Maximum Pain Relief with Your TENS Unit

Easy, Drug-Free Techniques for Treating Chronic Pain, Muscle Injuries, and Common Ailments at Home

Doctor Jo, PT, DPT

ULYSSES PRESS

Published in the United States by:
Ulysses Press
P.O. Box 3440
Berkeley, CA 94703
www.ulyssespress.com

ISBN13: 978-1-61243-937-2
Library of Congress Control Number 2019942127

Printed in the United States by Versa Press
10 9 8 7 6 5 4 3 2 1

Acquisitions editor: Casie Vogel
Managing editor: Claire Chun
Editor: Renee Rutledge
Proofreader: Jessica Benner
Design and production: what!design @ whatweb.com
Photographs: © Ask Doctor Jo, LLC

TENS unit devices and associated logos are owned by HealthmateForever and are used with permission.

Contents

Introduction

Electrical stimulation has been used for pain control in one form or another for centuries. There is even evidence that medical practitioners in ancient Rome had people stand on electric fish on the seashore to help relieve pain. Sounds a little fishy to me, but if it helped, who am I to judge?

Actual devices with static currents were used throughout the eighteenth century for general pain and headaches, but it wasn't until the early 1970s that the portable TENS (transcutaneous electrical nerve stimulation) unit was invented by American neurosurgeon C. Norman Shealy.

Known for his pain management and holistic therapies, Shealy graduated from the Duke University School of Medicine. In addition to the TENS device, he developed other spinal cord therapies in the early 1970s. Shortly after his success, many other companies began making similar TENS units of their own. The device was patented in 1974.

TENS units now range from very simple devices with preset settings to units that allow you to dial in specific parameters. They also vary greatly in size. Some are about the size of a remote control, while others fit in the palm of your hand. Some units can be controlled by your smartphone using Bluetooth technology. Others are rechargeable, have touch screens, or even have wireless electrodes. The available features and customizations now rival those of any electronic portable device.

Today's TENS units, however, didn't gain widespread popularity until 2014, shortly after the FDA started allowing them to be purchased over the counter. When this happened, the price of the units dropped significantly, and people quickly began to realize that these inexpensive units could help decrease acute and chronic pain while significantly reducing, or even eliminating, the need for often-dangerous medication.

In 2018, the Centers for Disease Control (CDC) analyzed 2016 National Health Interview Survey (NHIS) data. It found that an estimated 20.4 percent of US adults (about 50 million people) had chronic pain, and 8 percent of US adults (almost 20 million people) had high-impact chronic pain. Some research suggests that these numbers are actually much higher, with more than 100 million people affected by chronic pain, and this is just in the US.

Chronic pain can really take a toll physically and mentally. It can cause people to become depressed, lose their jobs, become addicted to pain killers, and suffer a higher risk of suicide. While there are no exact numbers for suicides and attempted suicides due to chronic pain, many doctors and experts believe they're much higher than we think.

Another big contributor to the rise in popularity of the TENS unit is the opioid epidemic. To help combat chronic pain, medical doctors often prescribe opioids as the first method of treatment, but some studies show opioids are helpful only about 50 percent of the time, and they come with many dangerous side effects. Long-term use of opioids builds up tolerance to the drugs, meaning stronger doses or more pills are needed to get the same effect. This can lead to addiction, overdoses, and even death.

Luckily, TENS and electrical muscle stimulation (EMS) units can help relieve chronic and acute pain without the dangerous side effects of medication. And while there are still conflicting studies about exactly how effective these units are when used over the long term, I've seen patients using a TENS unit in conjunction with stretches and exercises experience relief from both short-term acute pain and long-term chronic pain.

In this book, I mainly discuss TENS units. Most portable units today have a TENS/EMS combination. I talk about EMS in general terms, so you have a better understanding of your unit as a whole. (I will cover the specific qualities of TENS and EMS units, and the differences between them, in Chapter 2.) Even though TENS and EMS are different, both help with the healing process.

Who Am I?

Why should you care about what I have to say about TENS and EMS units?

First, let me share a bit about my background. I am a licensed physical therapist and a doctor of physical therapy. I graduated from PT school at the University of South Carolina in 2007. I have worked in many different settings, including outpatient, sports medicine, acute care, aquatics, and inpatient rehabilitation in both private and hospital-based clinics. I work with a wide variety of patients ranging in age from 1 to 92, including NFL athletes and great-great grandmothers.

You may recognize me from my Ask Doctor Jo YouTube channel, AskDoctorJo.com, and other social media channels where I have hundreds of thousands of subscribers.

Through these platforms, I show people the benefits of physical therapy. And if you've seen me online, then you probably know my pups love to make cameos in my videos and posts because, honestly, don't dogs always make things better?

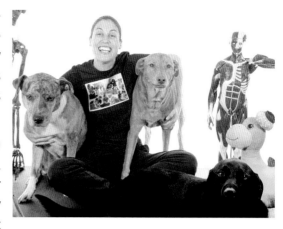

Growing up and in college, I played soccer. I was also a goalkeeper so, needless to say, I had many injuries throughout my soccer career. I have had a lot of physical therapy and, unfortunately, many orthopedic surgeries. The good thing is this allows me to easily relate to and empathize with my patients. With all my past injuries and surgeries, TENS/EMS units played a key role in my rehabilitation.

What to Expect

The goal of this book is to show you that TENS and EMS units can be a safe, noninvasive, user-friendly, and inexpensive way to help treat chronic and acute pain. In addition to showing you how to use a TENS/EMS unit, I'll also show you some simple stretches and exercises you can use in conjunction with the unit to get the best possible long-term results.

But before we dive into how to use TENS and EMS units for pain relief, it's important to know what pain is and why you are hurting. Often, once you know these two things, you can truly start to heal.

General Anatomy Terms

Here are some general anatomy terms you will see in this book.

Transcutaneous—Existing, applied, or measured across the depth of the skin.

Anterior—Nearer the front; especially situated in the front of the body or closer to the head.

Posterior—Farther back in position; of or closer to the rear or hind end of the body.

Medial—Pertaining to the middle; in or toward the middle; closer to the middle of the body.

Lateral—The side of the body or a body part that is farther from the middle or center of the body.

Sprain—Also known as a torn ligament. It is damage to one or more ligaments in a joint.

Strain—An injury to a muscle and/or tendon in which the muscle or tendon tears as a result of overstretching.

Contraindications—A condition or factor in which you should withhold a certain medical treatment due to the harm that it would or could cause.

Lumbar—Refers to the abdominal segment of the torso between the diaphragm and the sacrum. This region is sometimes referred to as the lower spine, or more generally, the low back.

Thoracic—Relating to the thorax, the part of the body between the neck and the abdomen.

Cervical—Relating to the neck.

Abduction (abduct)—The movement of a limb or other body part away from the midline of the body, or from another body part.

Adduction (adduct)—The movement of a limb or other body part toward the midline of the body or toward another body part.

Isometric exercise—Isometric exercise or isometrics are a type of strength training in which the joint angle and muscle length do not change during contraction.

Supine—Lying on your back or with your face upward.

Prone—Lying on your stomach or with your face downward.

Chapter 1

Different Kinds of Pain

What Is Pain?

So, what exactly is pain? This question is not as easy to answer as you might think. Pain, put quite simply, is your body's way of telling you something is wrong. Even though pain is not something you ever want to go through, it can literally save your life. Pain can also prevent you from making an injury or ailment worse because, if something hurts, you often slow down and try to figure out what is going on.

On the other hand, pain can also take away your quality of life. It can literally stop you in your tracks. It can prevent you from doing the things you enjoy, it can make you less productive at work or at home, and it can even leave you feeling frustrated and depressed. However, you should not suffer forever because of pain. If your doctor is telling you, "Sorry, there is nothing I can do, you will just have to live with it," then it's time to get a second opinion.

The way you feel pain is a pretty complicated process. Pain is felt when signals are sent from the site of pain to your brain and then back to the area of pain. Yes, you read that correctly—you don't actually feel pain as soon as your tissue is injured. Even though the signal is fast, you don't feel or react to pain until your brain gets the signal and tells you what to do.

Think of when you get stung by a bee: It takes a second or two until you feel the stinging sensation. In those few seconds, your brain gets the signal, processes it, and sends back a signal saying, "This hurts really badly, run!" or, "This only hurts a little. No need to panic, just swat that bee away." Then, your skin gets red and sometimes swelling (inflammation) occurs. The severity of your reaction completely depends on your brain, and different people can react very differently to that sting. One person might be allergic to bees and have a really bad reaction, while someone else might just have a little stinging sensation with no swelling at all.

To put things more technically, you have pain receptors throughout your body called nociceptors. When you encounter a noxious stimulus (a painful sensation), those receptors send an electrical impulse to the nerves where the injury is, and this signal then travels to the spinal cord. At the spinal cord, the signal can be heightened or decreased through a "gate" (I will talk more about this in the next chapter), and then it is sent to the brain. The brain then processes the information. It will decide things like how bad the pain is, where the pain is, and how to get away from the pain if necessary. After all that happens in the brain, the signal is sent back to the spinal cord, and you react to the pain. Whew! That's a lot going on in such a short period of time, and that's not even the whole process. It is much more complicated, but this gives you a general idea of what is happening.

Another word you might have heard before in relation to pain is neurotransmitters. These are chemicals in the nervous system that talk to each other to activate receptors. The activated receptors either block the pain or open like a gate to let the pain signals move through the body. This is how you perceive pain. Sometimes, though, there is a miscommunication with the signals, causing the gate to get stuck in the open position, and the pain becomes constant. This is chronic pain.

Certain medications, including opioids, have been created to decrease or block these signals so you don't feel as much pain. Your body also has the ability to produce natural opioid compounds such as endorphins. Endorphins are often released during exercise or things you enjoy, like eating chocolate, laughing, etc. These chemicals give you that happy feeling, or feeling of well-being. The opioids produced in our bodies are much stronger and more effective than any medication made.

Another reaction to pain is inflammation. Inflammation comes from the link between your nervous system and your immune system. But inflammation isn't always a bad thing. It's actually a good thing when it works like it's supposed to work. Inflammation helps to fight disease and heal injured tissue. The problem comes when it persists for long periods of time. Sometimes inflammation sticks around long after the tissue is healed, or sometimes signals get crossed and it will show up when there was never an injury to begin with. This can have a harmful effect on the tissue and can contribute to chronic pain.

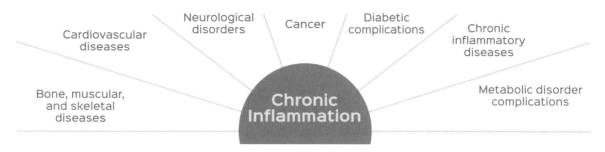

Chronic inflammation can lead to chronic pain and other diseases and disorders.

Often when I ask a patient, "What kind of pain are you having?" their reply is, "I don't know, it just hurts!" I agree, sometimes it is really hard to describe the type of pain you are having, but the way you "feel" the pain usually indicates what exactly is injured, like muscles, bones, nerves, etc. That's why healthcare providers always ask those types of questions.

In fact, when you are in a healthcare provider's office for the first time, you will most likely have to fill out a questionnaire about your pain. There's usually a list of words you can circle, such as sharp, dull, achy, shooting, numbness, tingling, throbbing, and constant. Trying to classify the type of pain you are having can definitely be overwhelming when you are hurting, but it really does make a difference because different types of pain usually "feel" differently.

Nociceptive Pain	Neuropathic Pain	Psychogenic Pain
• Dull • Achy • Throbbing • Tender to the touch • Hurts with movement	• Numbness • Tingling • Pins and needles • Shooting • Sharp • Electric • Constant	• Hard to pinpoint • Constant • Referred pain • Anxious

The way pain feels can indicate the type of pain you are experiencing. There are three main types of pain: nociceptive pain, neuropathic pain, and psychogenic pain. Let's explore each type.

Nociceptive Pain

Nociceptive pain is caused by damage to your skin, muscles, bones, or any other tissues in your body. This is the most common type of pain people experience, often described as dull, achy, or throbbing. Nociceptive pain can be caused by burns, cuts, sprains, strains, fractures, bruises, or other orthopedic injuries. This type of pain is very localized to one area, and it can be tender to the touch. It often hurts more with movement, and it can often feel better with rest, ice, compression, and elevation (RICE).

Neuropathic Pain

Neuropathic pain is caused by damage to the nerves. This is often a shooting, burning, numb, or tingling pain. Think of a time when your arm or leg "fell asleep." Maybe you slept on your arm funny, and when you woke up you couldn't move it. At first, it felt numb, then it felt tingly, maybe with a "pins and needles" sensation. Then you shook it, and the feeling slowly came back. Neuropathic pain is similar, but it lasts for a much longer period of time because nerves are very fragile vessels and heal at a much slower rate than other tissues in the body. Some of the main causes of neuropathic pain are diabetes, peripheral neuropathy, multiple sclerosis (MS), spinal surgeries and injuries, nerve compression from herniated discs or arthritis in the spine (sciatica), and chemotherapy. This type of pain is often constant, but can include sudden shooting or sharp pain. You can also experience significant pain with light pressure from touching the area or even clothing.

Psychogenic Pain

Affected by psychological factors, psychogenic pain consists of physical pain such as headaches, stomachaches, and even general back pain, but there's usually no physical injury or trauma. Instead it's caused by emotional, mental, and behavioral factors. Psychogenic pain can be brought on by big life events such as a death in the family, a breakup with a loved one, or even general anxiety. This type of pain is often difficult to pinpoint. There is an overall deep and aching feeling. It's usually constant, and there are areas of referred pain (where you perceive pain in an area, but the pain stimulus is somewhere else).

Acute Pain vs. Chronic Pain

In addition to the three different types of pain, the length of time you have the pain is broken into two different categories: acute pain and chronic pain. Though some definitions vary, acute pain usually lasts anywhere from three to six months, whereas chronic pain lasts longer than six months.

Acute pain usually happens suddenly and for a known reason. It is usually caused by a specific trauma, disease, or some sort of inflammation, and the pain will go away once the tissue is healed properly. Most of the time, acute pain is easily diagnosed by a healthcare professional and treated quickly.

Chronic pain can sometimes persist for years, long after the injured tissue is healed. Many forms of chronic pain involve an area that is constantly inflamed.

One of the most common types of inflammation-related chronic pain is arthritis. Arthritis can happen anywhere in the body, including the back, neck, hands, hips, and knees. Another very common type of chronic pain is general back pain. Approximately one-third of patients with low back pain develop persistent pain that lasts more than a year. Other common causes of back pain are spondylosis (degenerative changes in the spine), spondylolisthesis (slipping of the vertebra), herniated discs, and fibromyalgia.

It is not clearly understood why acute pain sometimes develops into chronic pain. Some research suggests it is caused by a "miscommunication" between your brain and the injured area, while other studies point to different factors. These include not allowing the injury to heal properly, not getting the best treatment for it, genetics, and the list goes on. No matter the cause of chronic pain, it can often be cured, reduced, or at least managed properly, so seek help. Don't just live with the pain.

Now that you know more than you probably ever wanted to know about pain, let's talk about some ways to get rid of it. In addition to a good stretching and exercise program, another one of my favorite treatments is using a TENS/EMS unit to help control your pain, improve circulation, and retrain your muscles so you can do the stretches and exercises you need to do to feel better.

Chapter 2

What Are TENS and EMS?

Electrical stimulation (ES) is a term used to describe treatments that deliver electrical currents to the body for the purpose of pain relief and rehabilitation. There are many types of ES, including functional electrical stimulation (FES), high-voltage pulsed current (HVPC), interferential current (IFC), neuromuscular electrical stimulation (NMES), transcutaneous electrical nerve stimulation (TENS), and electrical muscle stimulation (EMS). Wow, that's a lot of abbreviations! And to make things even more complicated, some companies that sell ES units also use their own terminology or abbreviations to differentiate their units from others on the market. You might see them called EMS, NMES, MS (muscle stimulators), and possibly others. Since EMS is the most popular term used for electrical muscle stimulation, I use EMS throughout the book for consistency.

Many types of ES are used mostly in a clinical setting. For the purposes of this book, let's focus on the forms of ES that are also designed for in-home use, specifically TENS and EMS.

Many TENS units made today also include EMS capabilities, so when learning how to properly use a TENS/EMS unit, it's important to know the difference between these two types of ES and which type of stimulation should be used for which types of injuries or ailments.

What Is TENS?

TENS units are becoming a popular way to help relieve acute and chronic pain without the use of medication. Basically, the TENS current runs along the nerve pathways to close the gate where the pain signal comes through. This reduces the pain that is felt, and sometimes completely stops the sensation of pain for a short period of time. If you're looking for a more technical definition, try this: a TENS unit activates a complex neuronal network to reduce pain by activating descending inhibitory systems in the central nervous system to reduce hyperalgesia (increased sensitivity to pain).

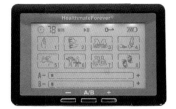

Theory Behind TENS

Earlier I explained how pain receptors send pain signals to the spinal cord via electrical impulses. Once those signals get to the spinal cord, they are basically in a holding station where a gate either opens and lets the pain signals pass to the brain or stays closed and stops the pain signal so you don't feel any pain at that time. Sometimes the signal gets through, but not completely, as though the gate is only partially open. So you will have pain, but it won't be as intense as the full signal. This phenomenon was first discovered by Ronald Melzack and Patrick D. Wall, who presented the gate control theory of pain in the 1960s. This theory is one of the main explanations as to why electrical stimulation like TENS works so well to control pain. The electrical current, like the body's electrical impulses, can close the gate to stop or decrease the pain signal to your brain.

Gate Control Theory of Pain

In 1965, Ronald Melzack and Patrick D. Wall introduced the gate control theory of pain in "Pain Mechanisms: A New Theory," published in *Science*. The theory transformed our understanding of pain mechanisms and management, explaining how the pain pathway works like a gate. The original theory has since been updated but still remains an important basis for understanding the complicated process of pain.

The gate control theory of pain was tested by Wall and William H. Sweet on eight patients with pain using high-frequency TENS. Even though the population size was small, their research published in 1967 did show patients reported pain relief during the stimulation and for about 30 minutes after the treatment.

Many researchers and clinicians believe there are other ways to open and close the gate to stop pain. Often, our emotions are a key factor, as explained in *Living a Healthy Life with Chronic Pain* by Sandra LeFort, MN, PhD, Lisa Webster, RN, et al.:

> *"Many factors can open or close the gate... For example, positive mood, distraction, and deep, relaxed breathing can act to close or partially close the gate while strong emotions like fear, anxiety, and expecting the worst can open the gate."*

I really like this explanation for a number of reasons—mainly because it addresses the ability to control the gate with your own thoughts. Even though some might not believe it's the case, having a positive attitude really can make a difference in how you feel. I see this time and time again with my patients. Those who have a positive outlook about their recovery tend to get better results than those who are pessimistic or negative. While this is not always the case, positivity helps.

How Does TENS Work?

We've talked about what TENS is, but how does TENS actually work? A TENS unit uses electrical currents that flow through electrodes placed on the skin to help control pain. Different frequencies, intensities, and durations can be used for different ailments. Studies show the frequencies activate central mechanisms in our bodies to produce analgesia, or a reduced feeling of pain. I will go into more detail about specific frequencies, settings, and how they are best used in Chapter 5.

What Is EMS?

Often, with an injury, your brain tells your muscles to go into protection mode by not contracting fully or, sometimes, not contract at all because the brain thinks this will cause further injury or pain. When this happens for a period of time, the muscles almost forget what they are supposed to do, and this often causes weakness and imbalances in the muscles. An EMS unit sends electrical impulses to the nerves, which makes the muscles contract. This forced contraction helps retrain the muscles by getting them to work the way they worked before the injury. It is important to note that EMS will not bulk you up or give you six-pack abs. It is specifically for retraining your muscles and helping them activate when they are not getting a full contraction on their own.

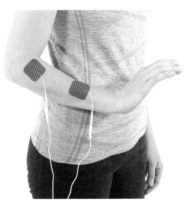

In this photo, the EMS unit is contracting the wrist extensor muscles, pulling the hand up.

The goal of EMS is to achieve a muscle contraction, whereas the goal of TENS is to achieve pain relief, but not a sustained muscle contraction.

How Does ES Help with Healing?

I often get asked, "Does TENS just help temporarily, or does it actually help with healing?" This is a great question, but you might get a different answer from each healthcare professional you ask. Research shows TENS and other ES help increase circulation to the area, and increased circulation helps the healing process. But I also believe if TENS helps reduce pain, then you are able to do the stretches and exercises you need to do to retrain your muscles, which helps with the healing. Less pain means more movement, which means improved healing.

Will a TENS/EMS Unit Work for Me?

As I mentioned in the introduction, I have experienced great results with TENS/EMS treatments for my patients, and I have also had fantastic results using the units for my own injuries and chronic pain. As an athlete growing up, I had many injuries that resulted in chronic pain and many orthopedic surgeries. With the use of TENS/EMS and physical therapy, I have been able to manage both acute pain and chronic pain with little to no pain medication.

With that said, most TENS/EMS studies on specific ailments are limited, and the parameters of these studies lack consistency. Therefore, the research is still mixed on how much TENS/EMS helps with chronic pain. Studies do show, however, that TENS/EMS can be very helpful with both acute and post-operative pain.

My own personal experiences and the positive studies that are available have led me to believe that TENS/EMS therapy can be very beneficial for pain management for a wide variety of common ailments and injuries. This is especially true when you combine TENS/EMS with other treatments like a healthy diet and a proper stretching and exercise program. Since TENS/EMS units are now very low cost and have little to no side effects, it is probably worth trying to see if it works for you. I'll show you some stretches and exercises you can do with your TENS/EMS unit for maximum, long-term pain relief in Chapter 9.

Do I Need a Prescription?

The short answer is no, but some insurance plans will cover the cost of a TENS/EMS unit if you have a prescription from your doctor. Units are very inexpensive and easy to get online or in some pharmacies without a prescription.

This was not the case when I first started as a physical therapist in 2007. Back then, TENS units were hundreds of dollars and difficult to get without a prescription. Some are very expensive, but they usually don't work any better than a $30 model. They just have more bells and whistles. I will go into more detail about different units in Chapter 4.

Chapter 3

Safety

Side Effects

The great thing about a TENS/EMS unit is there are very few side effects when it is used correctly. To be safe, make sure you are cleared by your healthcare professional to use one, and always follow the directions provided with your particular unit.

The biggest side effect you may encounter is a reaction to the electrode pads. Most electrodes have a sticky gel on the pads (or require you to apply a conductive gel), which might cause redness or irritation for some people. There is also the possibility of soreness or pain if you set the unit too high, and this can also cause redness and irritation where the pads are placed.

As with any medical device, it's important to remember there are many times you should NOT use the unit. I've listed some of the most universal precautions and contraindications for TENS/EMS units below, but every unit is different and may include additional precautions. Make sure you read through the specific precautions and contraindications of YOUR unit before using it.

Precautions and Contraindications

The precautions and contraindications for TENS units and EMS units are slightly different because an EMS unit produces a sustained contraction of the muscles. Precautions and contraindications for both unit types are listed here.

TENS Units
- Do not use if you have a pacemaker, defibrillator, or other electrical implant (it could damage the implant).

- Use during pregnancy only with your doctor's permission.

- Do not use on lower back or abdomen if pregnant.

- Do not use on any infected tissue or wounds.

- Do not use in areas where you think or know you have a malignancy (cancer).

- Do not use if you have an active deep vein thrombosis (DVT).

- Do not use if you have a hemorrhagic (bleeding) disorder.

- Do not use on neck or head area if you have seizures.

- Do not use on the chest area if you have heart issues.

- Do not use on genitalia.

- Do not use on the front of the neck or carotid area.

- Do not place on or cross over the eyes.

EMS Units

All of the TENS unit contraindications apply to EMS units as well. Here are some others:

- Do not use during pregnancy.

- Do not use on fractures or surgical sites that are unstable.

- Do not use on areas with osteoporosis.

- Do not use on areas with poor circulation.

- Do not use on chest muscles.

As with any treatment, some exceptions to the above precautions and contraindications apply but should be done ONLY if directed and supervised by your healthcare provider.

Cleaning Pads and Prepping Skin

To get the best performance out of your unit and the most longevity from your electrode pads, it's important to keep them clean and to properly prep your skin before applying them. Again, these are general instructions. Check the manual for your specific unit to see how to care for and apply your particular electrodes because they are all slightly different.

Each time you use a TENS/EMS unit, gently clean the skin where you are going to place the electrodes. You can use gentle soap and water or even just water. This will help remove some of your natural oils and other substances, like lotion, that decrease the stickiness of the electrodes. After washing your skin, make sure it is completely dry before applying the electrodes.

After each use, clean your electrodes with a wet, lint-free cloth (not a paper towel). It doesn't need much moisture, and sometimes just a few drops of water will be enough. Allow them to dry completely before your next use.

Some companies sell a spray or extra gel to help the electrode pads last longer, but, unfortunately, the pads will not last forever. If properly cared for, the pads can usually withstand 20 to 25 uses before they need to be replaced.

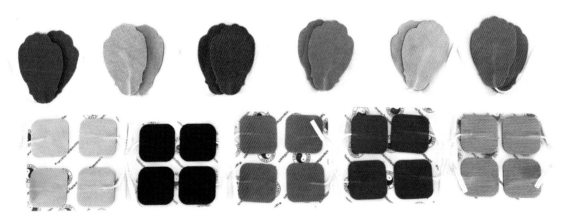

The most common sizes of electrodes are seen above.

Chapter 4

Units, Electrodes, and Channels

The TENS/EMS units available today range from very simple to very complex, and they also range from relatively inexpensive (at about $30) to $1,000 or more. With so many different models available, trying to figure out which one is the best for you can be overwhelming. I have reviewed and used many different brands. If you are interested in seeing the reviews, check out my website AskDoctorJo.com. My guidelines should be helpful as you research the best brand and unit for you.

Units—What Features Should I Get?

The first decision you'll want to make is whether you want just TENS or a unit that has both TENS and EMS functionality. Remember, TENS is for pain relief and should not cause a sustained muscle contraction, while EMS is for contracting the muscle to help rehab and retrain it. These are two very different currents, and you cannot substitute one for the other. If you think you will ever need EMS functionality,

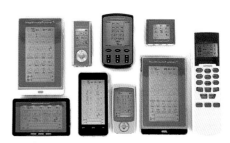

Units come in many shapes, sizes, and degrees of complexity.

then get a unit that does both. There is very little price difference between the two, and then you'll have the EMS option if you ever need it.

Once you've made that decision, the good news is that most units do the exact same thing—they deliver TENS and/or EMS currents. That's pretty much a given for all models (regardless of price or features) as long as you are purchasing it from a reputable company. Make sure you check the reviews! After that, you're basically paying for additional features. Think about buying a car. The base model will do the job of getting you from point A to point B, but there are lots of extra features you can add to make the car easier or more fun to drive.

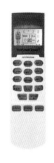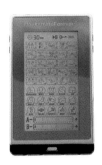

Purchase a unit with the features you think will benefit you the most. You want the unit's features to match your lifestyle. If you are confused by technology and purchase a unit that has so many advanced features you find it hard to use, you probably won't use it. On the other hand, if you love technology but get a basic unit, you may wish you had something with more bells and whistles.

A basic unit with few bells and whistles (left) and a more high-tech unit with many added features (right).

Whatever features you want, today's TENS/EMS units have you covered.

For general operations, there are simple units with big buttons you push to get the mode you want. (I will discuss modes further in the next chapter.) Units with LCD screens and rotary dials look a lot like the old iPods, and units with touch screens allow you to control everything by tapping the screen.

Units come in many different sizes (and colors), from something that can fit in the palm of your hand to something as big as a tablet. Most units are now rechargeable, but some use traditional AA or AAA batteries.

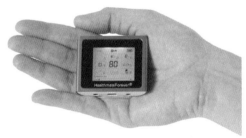

A unit small enough to fit in the palm of your hand.

Most units are also wired, meaning wires connect them to the electrodes, but there are wireless units, too. Wireless units usually cost more, but they allow you to move about more freely.

It doesn't stop there. Some units can be controlled by your smartphone, and others can even pulse to the beat of the music on your phone. There are many options to choose from, so make sure your unit has all the features you want. At the same time, don't pay for features you will never use.

Electrode Types

If your head isn't already spinning from all the unit options, the electrodes have almost as much variety as the units themselves. While all electrodes do the same thing (they deliver the current from the unit to the skin), all electrodes are not compatible with all units. As a result, it's important to know what types of electrodes can be used with your unit.

Electrodes typically come with one of two main connection types. The standard one is a pigtail type of pad where you push the cord prong into the pad. There are also pads that have button-type snaps, and these are becoming more popular. Be careful, because sometimes pads sold by one manufacturer don't always fit other brands, even if they appear to have the same type of connection. Get pads that are compatible with your unit's cords, or make sure they can be returned if they don't fit.

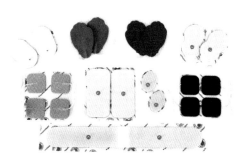

The colored electrodes have pigtail connections, and the white electrodes have button connections.

Electrodes also come in many different sizes. The standard size is 2" x 2", but a wide variety of additional sizes and shapes, from long and skinny to big and fat (the size of your hand), are available. Smaller pads work better for directing the current to a smaller, more specific spot, and larger ones work well for larger areas like the low back for general back pain.

Finally, most electrode pads now come pre-coated with a self-adhesive gel that is usually latex-free. As mentioned in the previous chapter, when cared for properly, these types of electrodes typically last for 20 to 25 uses. Some units still come with electrodes that require you to put your own gel on the pads. Usually these last longer, until the pads themselves crack or get holes in them. But these types of pads are not as common as they were in the past, since they do not stay in place as well as the self-adhesive ones.

Channels

There is also a component of TENS/EMS units called "channels." The following information about channels is specifically for wired units. Wireless units usually work a little differently. Even though they have channels, there is no physical connection, so make sure you read the unit's manual.

A channel controls the amount of current to the electrodes, and the current from the unit goes through the channel to the electrodes that are placed on your skin when you are using wires. Each channel has two electrodes that are connected to the channel with a single wire. Most simpler and traditional units have at least two channels, or what is sometimes called "dual" channels. Some units will have more.

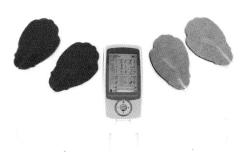

This unit has two channels with four electrodes.

Since each channel has two electrodes, if you use one channel you'll have two electrodes, and if you use two channels you'll have four electrodes. I will go into detail below about when to use one channel versus two.

Depending on your particular unit, some channels may be controlled together, while others may be controlled independently, so again, it's important to read your unit's manual to know how your channels are controlled. Channels that can be controlled independently are useful if you want to use each channel on a different area of the body at the same time. Or you can use independent channel control to make one pair of electrodes stronger than the other if you are using four electrodes in a crisscross pattern.

Chapter 5

Settings

Most TENS/EMS units today have preset modes. Depending on the unit, there can be anywhere from 3 to more than 24 different modes. Often they are labeled by body part, or even with a picture of the mode or type of current you should feel. Since all units are slightly different, read the manual for your specific unit to learn what the individual preset modes do.

For TENS/EMS combination units, some of the modes will be for TENS and some of the modes will be for EMS, although sometimes it's not clearly labeled which modes are for which type of current. Since TENS and EMS currents are intended for very different uses, make sure to read the unit's manual to know which is which.

Unfortunately, the manuals included with many of these units are not very clear, and some are also poorly translated from other languages. You may want to see if you can find a unit's manual online before purchasing it so you will know what you're getting as far as a manual and settings. This is especially important if you are purchasing a TENS/EMS combination unit, since you don't want to confuse a TENS setting for an EMS setting or vice versa.

It's important to know that even though some modes might be labeled for a particular ailment or injury, it's really about how it feels for you. Since a TENS unit is for pain control, you want to feel better when using it. So try the different modes to see which one you like best. What *you* think feels great might be very uncomfortable to me.

TENS is like any other treatment: when used long-term, you may build up a tolerance. If you feel like you are not getting as much relief after several uses, try a different mode or intensity to help prevent your body from adapting to the treatment. It's just like working out: you don't want to do the same workout every day or your muscles plateau, and you no longer get the most benefit from it.

Here are some of the most common preset modes you might find on a unit and what type of feeling they are meant to replicate. Your particular unit may have more or fewer preset modes.

Tui na is a type of alternative therapy used in traditional Chinese medicine. It often involves massage and acupressure, which is believed to open the flow of Qi, or energy in your body. Often shown as hands "massaging" the back, this setting simulates massage and can help with pain relief and relaxation.

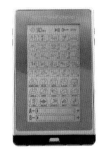

Preset modes can be helpful but are sometimes a little confusing.

Acupuncture is a form of traditional Chinese medicine that uses thin needles inserted to certain areas of the body to help correct imbalances through meridian channels, which are basically energy pathways throughout the body. Often shown as a hand with a needle, this mode provides the sensation of an acupuncture needle without the needle. It usually causes a quick, deep contraction.

Tapping is a technique that consists of tapping with the fingers along meridian points, which are specific points along the meridian channels, in an effort to energize the body. Often shown as a fist "tapping" up and down, this mode produces a thumping sensation that massages and helps relax your muscles.

Gua Sha is a form of traditional Chinese medicine that involves scraping the skin with a massage tool to improve circulation. Often shown as a hand with a stone-like tool, this mode simulates a scratching or kneading sensation with a low-frequency setting and is believed to help with stiffness and internal pain.

Cupping is a Chinese form of alternative medicine that involves suctioning an area of skin with a cup to increase blood flow. Shown as a hand with a cup, this mode simulates a sensation of suction on your skin, which can help increase circulation.

Shiatsu is an ancient Japanese therapy where pressure is applied with fingers and hands to acupressure sites. Often shown as a finger putting pressure on the body, this mode simulates a type of finger and palm pressure with massage.

Pressure is the technique of pushing hard to get a feeling of pressure on the skin. Often shown as two hands with their palms down and thumbs slightly together, this mode simulates a massage technique that can help relax superficial and deeper layers of muscle and connective tissue.

Deep tissue massage is a technique of using the elbow or a tool to get to deeper tissue. Often shown as an elbow pushing into the body, this mode simulates a deep tissue massage, which can help relieve chronic muscle tension.

Bodybuilding is a setting for muscle retraining. Often shown as two dumbbells, this mode strengthens and tones the muscles to some extent, or retrains muscles.

Combination usually consists of multiple techniques combined. Often shown as two yin and yang signs, this mode is a random combination of the other modes listed above.

In addition to these preset modes, some units also have modes that are designed for a specific body part. Sometimes you will see settings for the knee, ankle, back, etc. As I mentioned earlier, these presets are a good place to start, but, ultimately, you should use the setting that feels the best to you and provides the most pain relief.

Intensity: How Strong Should It Be?

Once you select the mode you want to use, the next step on most units is to set the intensity, or how strong or weak to deliver the current. Again, you are going for comfort and pain relief here, so the intensity should be strong, but it should *never* hurt.

The intensity also depends on whether or not you get a contraction. In general, with a TENS unit, you should not get a contraction for a sustained period of time. Some settings (like the acupuncture setting) will create a quick contraction to help relax the muscle. However, if you are getting a strong muscle contraction with the TENS unit, you have the intensity too high, or you might need to adjust your electrode placements.

Duration: How Long Should It Be On?

Most units allow you to set a timer for the duration you want the unit to function. After the time is up, the unit turns off. Most timers include a range of 10 to 80 minutes. On average, you want to use a TENS unit for only 15 to 30 minutes. With longer times, your body can start to adapt to the stimulation, which will reduce its effectiveness.

If you are using a stronger intensity, or a mode like acupuncture that causes quick muscle contractions, you probably want to set the timer for even less time so your muscles don't fatigue. For more information on specific mode times, see the table on page 25.

For EMS, you should use the unit for only about 5 to 10 minutes at a time. Since the muscles contract for a longer amount of time with EMS, you want to fatigue muscles to work them, but don't over fatigue (or exhaust) injured muscles.

Frequency: How Often Should I Use It?

Generally, you can use any of the modes one to five times a day, but this depends on your specific injury, how long you have had that injury, and your tolerance to the electrical stimulation. So it's always best to ask what your healthcare provider recommends for your particular situation.

Traditional Settings

Technical alert! If you have a preset TENS unit and don't like technical jargon, feel free to skip this section.

Since most units today come with preset modes like the ones described on page 22, you don't have to worry as much about how to set your unit. However, if you have a traditional TENS unit where you have to set your own parameters, if you are a techie person and like to know how things work, or if you just like having more control over your treatment, this section is for you.

With a traditional TENS unit, different TENS settings can be used, including the conventional (normal) TENS, acupuncture-like TENS, and intense TENS. For these units, you can adjust the pulse amplitude, frequency, width (or duration), and pattern of the currents for different end goals, as shown in the table on page 25.

The variables on TENS units differ slightly, but most fall in these ranges:

- Output intensity: 0 to 100 mA
- Pulse frequency: 2 to 150 pps or Hz
- Pulse width: 50 to 250 μs

There are three modes: normal, burst, and modulation, which are used with the above settings to regulate the pulses or pattern of the current. The burst and modulation modes help minimize the chance of your body adapting to the current, which decreases the analgesia effect. There are no parameters for these modes; you pick the mode you want with the setting you want.

Normal mode is a constant pulse of the parameters you set in the unit. This is usually more comfortable, but your body can adapt to it quickly and build up a tolerance to the pulses.

Burst mode is just like it sounds. The pulse comes out in bursts, usually two to three bursts per second.

Modulation mode is a more irregular mode, which helps prevent the body from building up a tolerance to the pulses.

	Conventional (Normal) TENS	Acupuncture-like TENS	Intense TENS
Intensity or Pulse Amplitude (mA or milliampere)*	Low: strong, comfortable, non-painful paresthesia	High: hyperstimulation, non-painful muscle twitches	High: referred pain analgesia, blocks peripheral nerves
Frequency (hertz), Pulse Rate (pulse per second)	High: 50 to 100 Hz, 80 to 100 pps	Low: 2 to 4 Hz, 100 to 200 pps	High: 50 to 120 Hz, up to 200 pps
Pulse Duration or Pulse Width (microsecond)	Small pulse width: 50 to 200 µs	Longer pulse width: 150 to 400 µs	Longer pulse width: 200 µs or higher
What Should I Feel?	Strong but comfortable tingling or prickly feeling	Strong but comfortable quick muscle contractions	Very uncomfortable tingling or prickly feeling. As strong as you can tolerate
What Is It Used For?	Most commonly used setting for pain; stops nerve pain	Use over acupuncture points, trigger points, or sore muscles	Blocks peripheral nerves and referred pain; rapid pain relief
How Often and for How Long Should I Use It?	15 to 30 minutes per session; up to five times a day	15 to 20 minutes per session; up to three times a day	A few minutes at a time, 10 minutes at most; one to two times a day

* Intensity varies throughout the treatment, and it will be different from person to person. You can slowly increase the intensity as your body adapts to the current throughout the treatment.

Chapter 6

Electrode Placements for TENS

In this chapter and the ones that follow, all photos will show electrode pad placements with different-colored electrode pads representing each channel (typically, red for channel A and blue for channel B). This will help you see how each channel is being placed. Remember, wired units have two electrodes for each channel. Some wireless units, however, have a single pad for each channel. If this is the case with your wireless pads, refer to Chapter 8, Electrode Placements for Wireless Units.

Quick tip: if you are using the electrodes on an area that is hairy, you may want to shave that area to get the best conductivity. This will also help keep the electrodes cleaner, so you can use them longer before they'll need replacing. And, maybe even more importantly, it will prevent the painful pull of hair when you remove the pad!

For a TENS unit, you can use one channel (two electrodes) or two channels (four electrodes). Both are effective, so I usually decide based on the size of the area of pain I'm trying to cover. The general rule is, if you want a very specific area to get the current, like a trigger point or a smaller area like your wrist or elbow, you should use one channel. Place the two electrodes on either side of the spot of pain since the current runs back and forth between electrodes.

Four electrodes is a better choice for a more general area of pain like low back pain or quadriceps pain. The key point to remember with four electrodes is the two channels need to cross like an X with the main area of pain in the middle of the X (X marks the spot). This is often not explained in the instruction manual and can affect the intensity and benefits you feel at the site of pain.

While the placement of electrodes for TENS is typically at the site of the pain or injury, they do not have to be exact as long as you are getting pain relief. You may have to move the electrodes around a few times before you find the best placement for pain relief. If you need to move the electrodes, turn off the unit (or pause the unit if yours has a pause feature) before moving the electrodes. Often you will feel the current more strongly in one area than

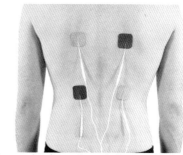

Channel A is red, and channel B is blue. They cross with an X pattern to cover the full pain area of the mid back.

another, so pausing or turning off the unit ensures you don't get more intensity than you want. It also prevents the current from running into your fingers while you move the electrodes, which can be an unpleasant feeling.

Now I will show you specific electrode placements on different areas of the body. Each section is broken down to a specific area of the body along with common ailments that are alleviated by those placements. There are no placements shown on the chest area because it is contraindicated if you have heart issues.

GENERAL KNEE PAIN

Channels: 2

Method: TENS

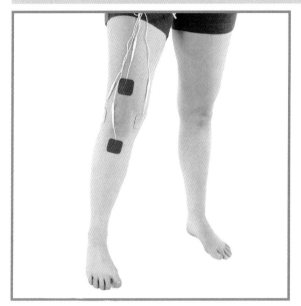 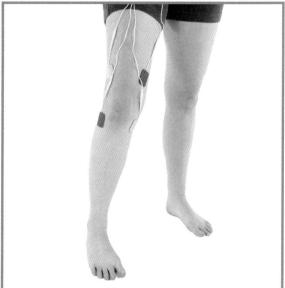

Use two-channel placements for a larger or general area of knee pain. For the wired units, each channel has two electrodes as shown above. Channel A is depicted with the red electrodes, and channel B is depicted with the blue electrodes.

Use an X pattern for the placements, crossing the channels over the general area of pain.

These placements can be used for a number of injuries and ailments, including but not limited to: general knee pain, knee tendonitis, knee bursitis, plica syndrome, anterior cruciate ligament (ACL) tear/sprain, meniscus injury or tear, patellofemoral pain syndrome (PFPS), chondromalacia patella (runner's knee), knee osteoarthritis or arthritis, medial collateral ligament (MCL) tear/sprain, posterior cruciate ligament (PCL) tear/sprain, lateral collateral ligament (LCL) tear/sprain, patellar tendonitis, total knee arthroplasty (TKA) or total knee replacement (TKR), and other post-surgery pain.

MEDIAL KNEE PAIN

Channels: 1

Method: TENS

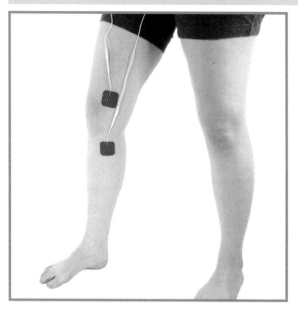 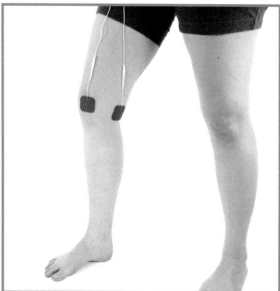

On smaller or more specific areas of the medial knee, use one channel with two electrodes to more easily get the placements you want. Make sure the area of pain is in between the two electrodes.

These placements can be used for a number of injuries and ailments of the medial knee, including but not limited to: pes anserine bursitis, MCL injury, and medial meniscal tear.

LATERAL KNEE PAIN

Channels: 1

Method: TENS

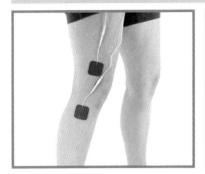 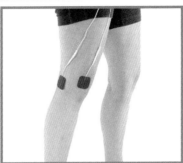 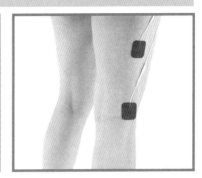

On smaller or more specific areas of the lateral knee, use one channel with two electrodes to more easily get the placements you want. Make sure the area of pain is in between the two electrodes.

These placements can be used for a number of injuries and ailments of the lateral knee, including but not limited to: LCL injury, iliotibial (IT) band syndrome, and lateral meniscal tear.

HAMSTRING STRAIN

Channels: 1

Method: TENS

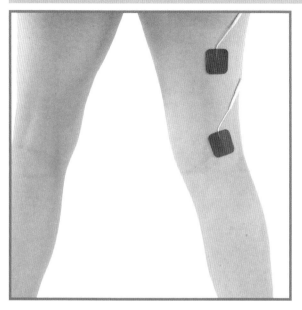

On smaller or more specific areas like along the hamstrings behind the knee, use one channel with two electrodes to more easily get the placements you want. Make sure the area of pain is in between the two electrodes.

PATELLAR TENDONITIS
(Jumper's Knee)

Channels: 1

Method: TENS

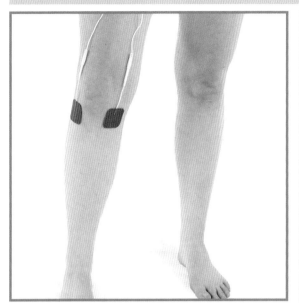 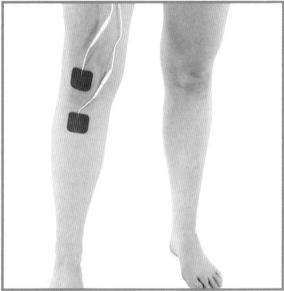

On smaller or more specific areas like the patellar tendon, use one channel with two electrodes to more easily get the placements you want. Make sure the area of pain is in between the two electrodes.

QUADRICEPS STRAIN

Channels: 1 or 2

Method: TENS

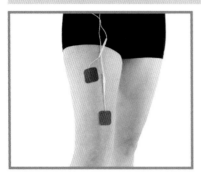 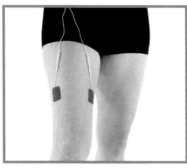 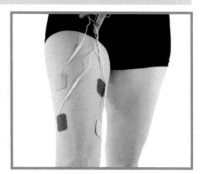

On smaller or more specific areas like on the quadriceps, use one channel with two electrodes to more easily get the placements you want. Make sure the area of pain is in between the two electrodes.

If the area of pain in the quadriceps is more general and covers a larger area, consider using two channels with four electrodes. Make sure the channels cross the area of pain.

LOWER LEG PAIN

Channels: 1 or 2

Method: TENS

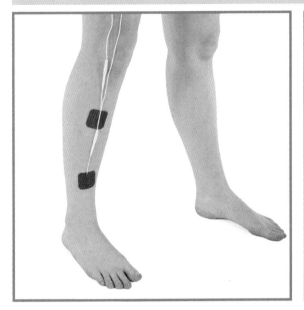
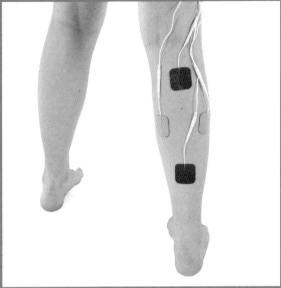

In the photos above, channel A is depicted with the red electrodes, and channel B is depicted with the blue electrodes. Depending on the size of the area of pain, you can use one channel (two electrodes) or two channels (four electrodes) around the area of pain.

For a larger or general area of pain, use two channels, crossing them in an X pattern over the general area of pain.

These placements can be used for a number of injuries and ailments, including but not limited to: general leg pain, calf strain, and anterior shin splints.

GENERAL ANKLE PAIN

Channels: 2

Method: TENS

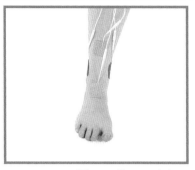 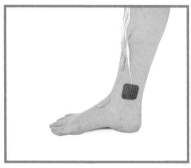 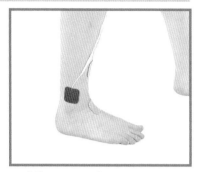

These three pictures show a four-electrode placement at different angles.

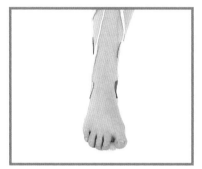 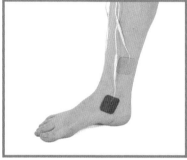 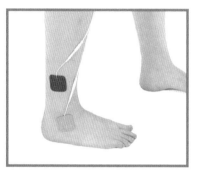

Alternate placement: These three pictures show a four-electrode placement at different angles.

Use two-channel placements for a larger or general area of pain. For the wired units, each channel has two electrodes as shown above. Channel A is depicted with the red electrodes, and channel B is depicted with the blue electrodes.

Use an X pattern for the placements, crossing the channels over the general area of pain.

These placements can be used for a number of injuries and ailments, including but not limited to: ankle sprain, ankle arthritis, ankle tendonitis, tarsal tunnel syndrome, posterior shin splints, medial ankle sprain, peroneal tendonitis, and lateral ankle sprain.

MEDIAL ANKLE PAIN

Channels: 1

Method: TENS

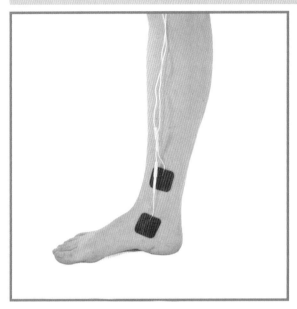 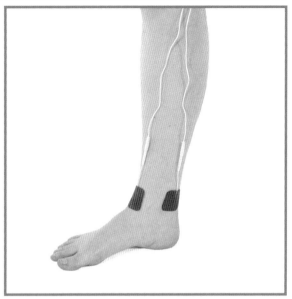

On smaller or more specific areas of the medial ankle, use one channel with two electrodes to more easily get the placements you want. Make sure the area of pain is in between the two electrodes.

These placements can be used for a number of injuries and ailments of the medial ankle, including but not limited to: tarsal tunnel syndrome, posterior shin splints, distal tibia fractures, and medial ankle sprain.

LATERAL ANKLE PAIN

Channels: 1

Method: TENS

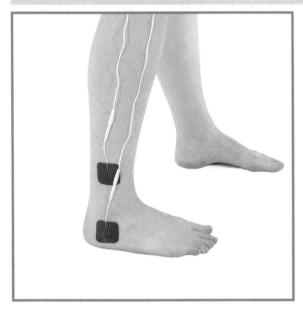 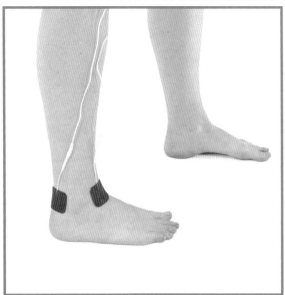

On smaller or more specific areas of the lateral ankle, use one channel with two electrodes to more easily get the placements you want. Make sure the area of pain is in between the two electrodes.

These placements can be used for a number of injuries and ailments of the lateral ankle, including but not limited to: peroneal tendonitis, fibular fractures, and lateral ankle sprain.

FOOT PAIN

Channels: 2

Method: TENS

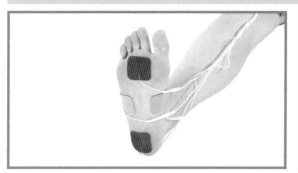 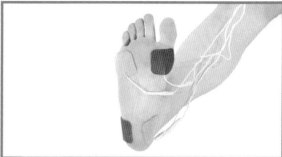

For pain on the plantar (bottom) surface of the foot.

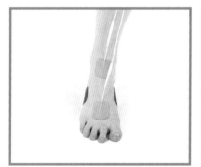 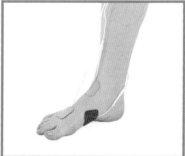 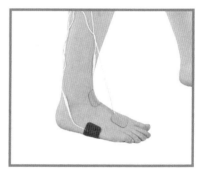

These three pictures show a four-electrode placement at different angles for the foot.

Use two-channel placements for a larger or general area of pain. For the wired units, each channel has two electrodes as shown above. Channel A is depicted with the red electrodes, and channel B is depicted with the blue electrodes.

Use an X pattern for the placements, crossing the channels over the general area of pain.

This placement can be used for a number of injuries and ailments, including but not limited to: diabetic peripheral neuropathy, plantar fasciitis, foot drop, heel spurs, and foot arthritis.

HEEL PAIN

Channels: 1

Method: TENS

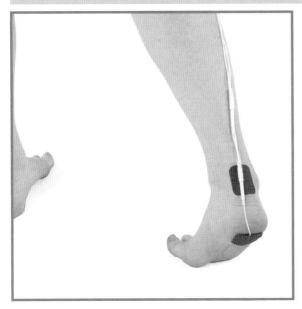

On smaller or more specific areas of the heel, use one channel with two electrodes to more easily get the placements you want. Make sure the area of pain is in between the two electrodes.

These placements can be used for a number of injuries and ailments of the heel, including but not limited to: heel spurs, Achilles tendonitis, foot arthritis, and calcaneus fracture.

GENERAL HIP PAIN

Channels: 2

Method: TENS

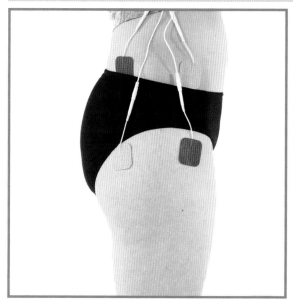

Use two-channel placements for a larger or general area of pain. For the wired units, each channel has two electrodes as shown above. Channel A is depicted with the red electrodes, and channel B is depicted with the blue electrodes.

Use an X pattern for the placements, crossing the channels over the general area of pain.

These placements can be used for a number of injuries and ailments, including but not limited to: hip osteoarthritis, hip tendonitis, hip bursitis, IT band syndrome, tensor fasciae latae (TFL) pain, and total hip joint replacement/arthroplasty (THR/THA).

LATERAL HIP PAIN

Channels: 1

Method: TENS

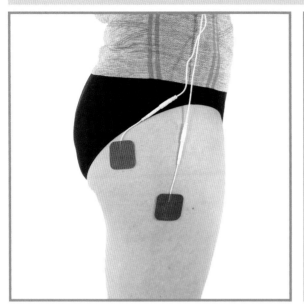 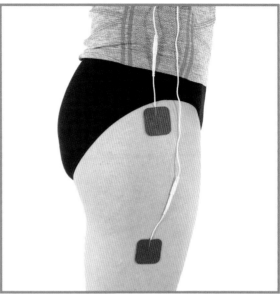

On smaller or more specific areas of the lateral hip, use one channel with two electrodes to more easily get the placements you want. Make sure the area of pain is in between the two electrodes.

These placements can be used for a number of injuries and ailments of the lateral hip, including but not limited to: greater trochanteric hip bursitis, TFL pain, piriformis syndrome, and IT band syndrome.

MEDIAL HIP (Inner Thigh) PAIN

Channels: 1

Method: TENS

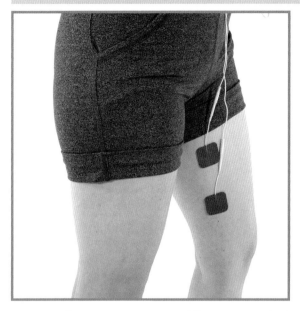

On smaller or more specific areas of the medial hip, use one channel with two electrodes to more easily get the placements you want. Make sure the area of pain is in between the two electrodes.

These placements can be used for a number of injuries and ailments of the medial hip, including but not limited to: femoroacetabular impingement (FAI), groin strain, hip labral tear/repair, adductor strain, and hip arthritis.

ANTERIOR HIP PAIN

Channels: 1

Method: TENS

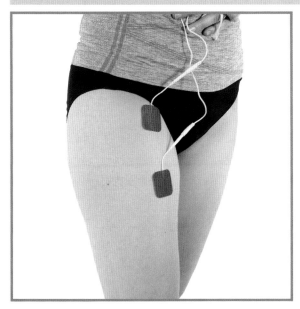

On smaller or more specific areas of the anterior hip, use one channel with two electrodes to more easily get the placements you want. Make sure the area of pain is in between the two electrodes.

These placements can be used for a number of injuries and ailments of the anterior hip, including but not limited to: hip flexor strain, hip flexor tendonitis, hip labral tear/repair, and hip arthritis.

POSTERIOR HIP PAIN

Channels: 1

Method: TENS

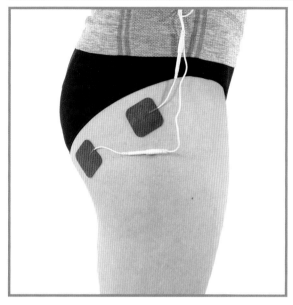

On smaller or more specific areas of the posterior hip, use one channel with two to more easily get the placements you want. Make sure the area of pain is in between the two electrodes.

These placements can be used for a number of injuries and ailments of the posterior hip, including but not limited to: hamstring strain, piriformis pain syndrome, gluteal strain, hip labral tear/repair, sciatica, and sacroiliac (SI) joint pain.

GENERAL LOW BACK (Lumbar) PAIN

Channels: 2

Method: TENS

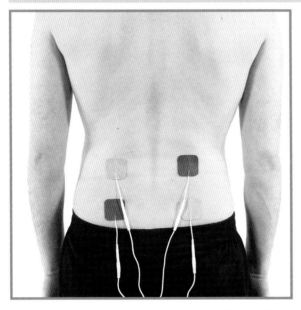

Use two-channel placements for a larger or general area of pain. For the wired units, each channel has two electrodes as shown above. Channel A is depicted with the red electrodes, and channel B is depicted with the blue electrodes.

Use an X pattern for the placements, crossing the channels over the general area of pain.

These placements can be used for a number of injuries and ailments, including but not limited to: degenerative disc disease (DDD), herniated disc pain, low back/lumbar pain/strain, SI joint pain, sciatica, fibromyalgia, and facet joint pain.

LOW BACK (Lumbar) PAIN—ONE SIDE

Channels: 1

Method: TENS

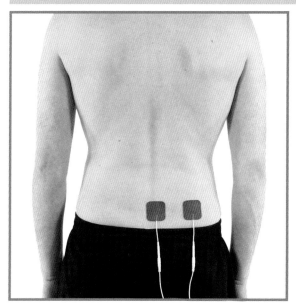 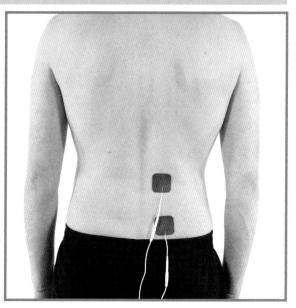

On smaller or more specific areas of the low back, use one channel with two electrodes to more easily get the placements you want. Make sure the area of pain is in between the two electrodes.

These placements can be used for a number of injuries and ailments of the low back, including but not limited to: SI joint pain, muscle strain, facet joint pain, and sciatica.

GENERAL MID TO UPPER BACK (Thoracic) PAIN (Two Channels)

Channels: 2

Method: TENS

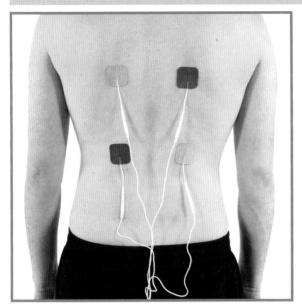 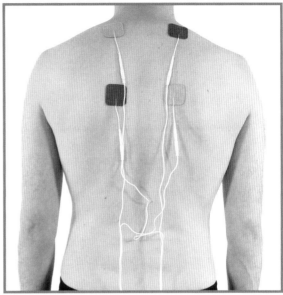

Use two-channel placements for a larger or general area of pain. For the wired units, each channel has two electrodes as shown above. Channel A is depicted with the red electrodes, and channel B is depicted with the blue electrodes.

Use an X pattern for the placements, crossing the channels over the general area of pain.

These placements can be used for a number of injuries and ailments, including but not limited to: DDD, herniated disc pain, upper back/thoracic pain/strain, latissimus dorsi (lat) strain, fibromyalgia, and rhomboid strain.

GENERAL MID TO UPPER BACK (Thoracic) PAIN (One Channel)

Channels: 1

Method: TENS

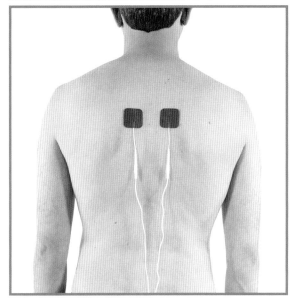

On smaller or more specific areas on the mid to upper back, use one channel with two electrodes to more easily get the placements you want. Make sure the area of pain is in between the two electrodes.

These placements can be used for a number of injuries and ailments of the mid to upper back, including but not limited to: rhomboid strain, middle trapezius pain, and thoracic back pain.

GENERAL NECK (Cervical) PAIN

Channels: 2

Method: TENS

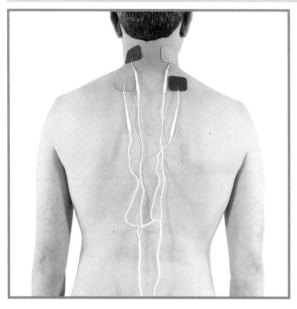

Use two-channel placements for a larger or general area of pain. For the wired units, each channel has two electrodes as shown above. Channel A is depicted with the red electrodes, and channel B is depicted with the blue electrodes.

Use an X pattern for the placements, crossing the channels over the general area of pain.

These placements can be used for a number of injuries and ailments, including but not limited to: cervicogenic headaches, DDD, herniated disc pain, migraine headaches, neck/cervical pain/strain, neck arthritis, fibromyalgia, and tension headaches.

GENERAL NECK (Cervical) PAIN (One Side)

Channels: 1

Method: TENS

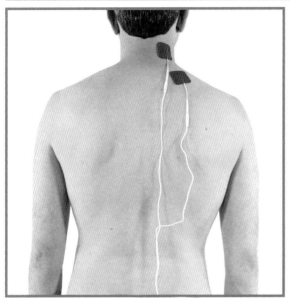

On smaller or more specific areas on the neck, use one channel with two electrodes to more easily get the placements you want. Make sure the area of pain is in between the two electrodes.

These placements can be used for a number of injuries and ailments of one side of the neck, including but not limited to: neck strain, upper trapezius (trap) pain, levator scapulae strain, scapula pain, and cervicogenic headaches.

GENERAL SHOULDER PAIN

Channels: 2

Method: TENS

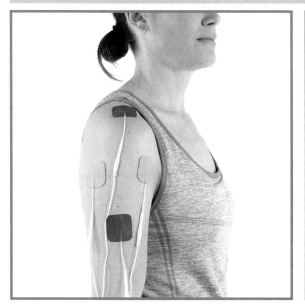 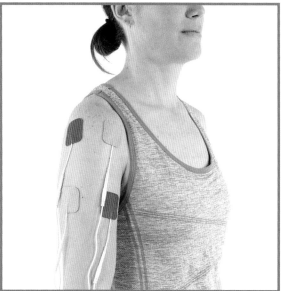

Use two-channel placements for a larger or general area of pain. For the wired units, each channel has two electrodes as shown above. Channel A is depicted with the red electrodes, and channel B is depicted with the blue electrodes.

Use an X pattern for the placements, crossing the channels over the general area of pain.

These placements can be used for a number of injuries and ailments, including but not limited to: frozen shoulder (adhesive capsulitis), shoulder labral tear/repair, total shoulder replacement/total shoulder arthroplasty (TSR/TSA), shoulder osteoarthritis, shoulder tendonitis, shoulder bursitis, shoulder impingement, subacromial bursitis, biceps tendonitis, acromioclavicular (AC) joint sprain, and rotator cuff tear/repair.

BICEPS TENDONITIS

Channels: 1

Method: TENS

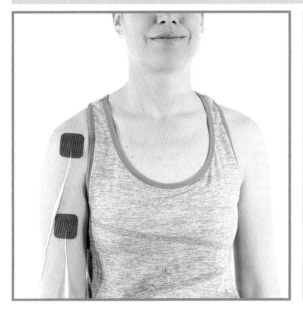 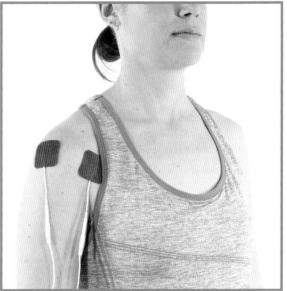

On smaller or more specific areas like the biceps tendon, use one channel with two electrodes to more easily get the placements you want. Make sure the area of pain is in between the two electrodes.

AC JOINT SPRAIN

Channels: 1

Method: TENS

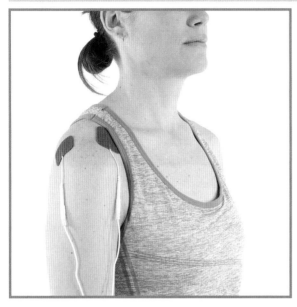

On smaller or more specific areas like the AC joint, use one channel with two electrodes to more easily get the placements you want. Make sure the area of pain is in between the two electrodes.

ROTATOR CUFF TEAR/REPAIR
(or Shoulder Impingement)

Channels: 1

Method: TENS

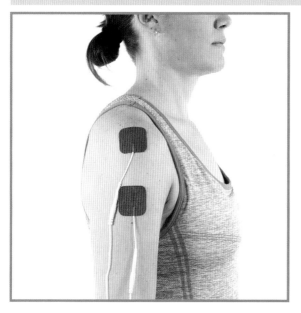

On smaller or more specific areas like the rotator cuff tendons, use one channel with two electrodes to more easily get the placements you want. Make sure the area of pain is in between the two electrodes.

GENERAL ELBOW PAIN

Channels: 2
Method: TENS

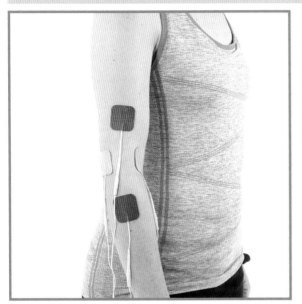 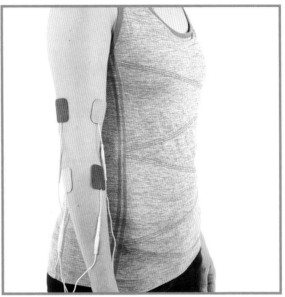

Use two-channel placements for a larger or general area of pain. For the wired units, each channel has two electrodes as shown above. Channel A is depicted with the red electrodes, and channel B is depicted with the blue electrodes.

Use an X pattern for the placements, crossing the channels over the general area of pain.

These placements can be used for a number of injuries and ailments, including but not limited to: cubital tunnel syndrome, medial epicondylitis (golfer's elbow), lateral epicondylitis (tennis elbow), elbow bursitis, and triceps tendonitis.

POSTERIOR ELBOW PAIN

Channels: 1

Method: TENS

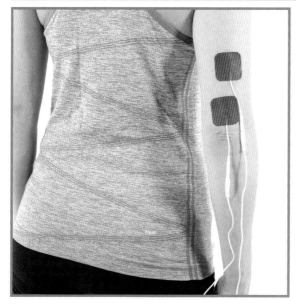

On smaller or more specific areas on the elbow, use one channel with two electrodes to more easily get the placements you want. Make sure the area of pain is in between the two electrodes.

These placements can be used for a number of injuries and ailments of the posterior elbow, including but not limited to: cubital tunnel syndrome, elbow bursitis, and triceps tendonitis.

ANTERIOR ELBOW PAIN

Channels: 1

Method: TENS

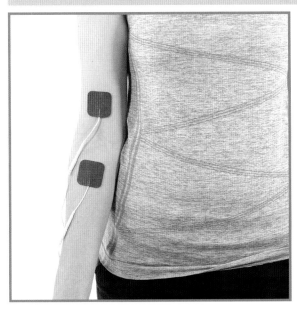

On smaller or more specific areas on the elbow, use one channel with two electrodes to more easily get the placements you want. Make sure the area of pain is in between the two electrodes.

These placements can be used for a number of injuries and ailments of the anterior elbow, including but not limited to: (distal) biceps tendonitis.

GOLFER'S ELBOW

Channels: 1

Method: TENS

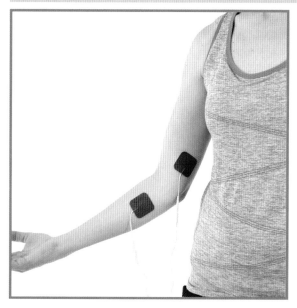

On smaller or more specific areas like the medial elbow, use one channel with two electrodes to more easily get the placements you want. Make sure the area of pain is in between the two electrodes.

TENNIS ELBOW

Channels: 1

Method: TENS

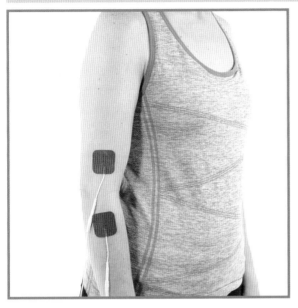

On smaller or more specific areas like the lateral elbow, use one channel with two electrodes to more easily get the placements you want. Make sure the area of pain is in between the two electrodes.

GENERAL WRIST PAIN (Two Channels)

Channels: 2

Method: TENS

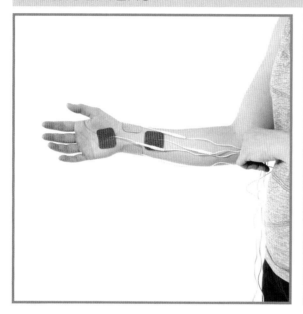 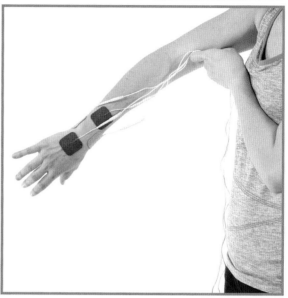

Use two-channel placements for a larger or general area of pain. For the wired units, each channel has two electrodes as shown above. Channel A is depicted with the red electrodes, and channel B is depicted with the blue electrodes.

Use an X pattern for the placements, crossing the channels over the general area of pain.

These placements can be used for a number of injuries and ailments, including but not limited to: wrist pain, carpal tunnel syndrome, wrist sprain, and wrist arthritis.

GENERAL WRIST PAIN (One Channel)

Channels: 1

Method: TENS

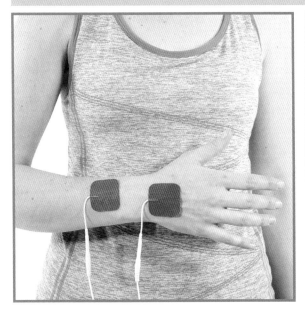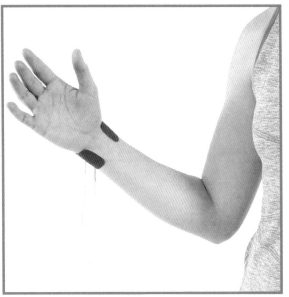

On smaller or more specific areas on the wrist, use one channel with two electrodes to more easily get the placements you want. Make sure the area of pain is in between the two electrodes.

These placements can be used for a number of injuries and ailments of the wrist, including but not limited to: wrist pain, carpal tunnel syndrome, wrist sprain, and wrist arthritis.

GENERAL HAND PAIN

Channels: 1

Method: TENS

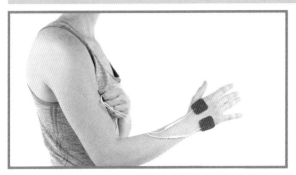

On smaller or more specific areas on the hand, use one channel with two electrodes to more easily get the placements you want. Make sure the area of pain is in between the two electrodes.

These placements can be used for a number of injuries and ailments of the hand, including but not limited to: diabetic peripheral neuropathy and rheumatoid arthritis (RA).

***

These miscellaneous ailments can come with large or specific areas of pain that may vary from person to person.

- Complex regional pain syndrome (CRPS)
- Reflex sympathetic dystrophy (RSD)
- Fibromyalgia
- Menstrual pain/cramping
- Multiple sclerosis (MS)
- Phantom limb pain
- Spinal cord injuries
- Stroke

So, depending on where you are feeling the pain, use the same placement guidelines for that area (back, neck, shoulder, etc.). If you want a more specific area, using one channel with two electrodes is best. If you want to cover a more general or larger area of pain, two channels with four electrodes will be best. And remember to always place the electrodes around the point of pain.

Chapter 7

Electrode Placements for EMS

Unlike a TENS electrode placement, an EMS electrode placement needs to be more specific and requires only one channel (two electrodes). Since EMS is used to get a sustained muscle contraction and retrain the muscle, the two electrodes should run along the muscle you wish to activate. If you were in a physical therapy clinic, the physical therapist might use probes that run along the surface to find the best spots for getting a muscle contraction, or even use their hands to feel for the muscle contraction. If you have not been to a healthcare provider to help you identify the best placement, you will need to use trial and error to get the best placement for the EMS electrodes. Once you find the placements that cause the muscle to contract, it will be easy to find those spots again in future sessions.

Remember, if you need to reposition the electrodes, turn the unit off (or pause the unit if it has a pause feature) before moving them.

I do not recommend using EMS for muscle contractions on areas near the spine, since crossing the spine would put the electrodes on different muscles that produce different movements. This could pull the spine out of alignment. I also do not recommend using an EMS for the chest area, since it is contraindicated to use it over the heart.

THE KNEE—QUADRICEPS (Quad) MUSCLE

Channels: 1

Method: EMS

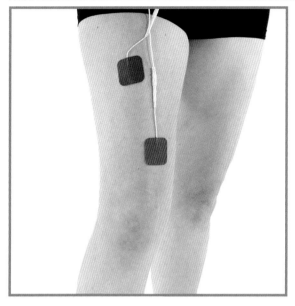

Place the electrodes along the quad muscle. This muscle helps extend or straighten the knee. It's very important in walking, running, jumping, and squatting, and can cause pain and instability in the knee when it's not working properly.

The goal of this placement is to contract and retrain the quad muscles. If your knee is bent, the contraction will straighten it out if it's strong enough, just as it would if you were actively contracting your quad muscles.

THE LOWER LEG/ANKLE/FOOT—ANTERIOR TIBIALIS MUSCLE

Channels: 1

Method: EMS

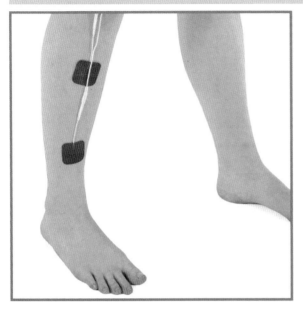

Place the electrodes along the anterior tibialis muscle (or tibialis anterior muscle). This muscle helps dorsiflex (pull up) your foot when walking. If this muscle is not working properly, it can cause difficulty walking (drop foot), injuries to your ankle (ankle sprains), and possible falls.

The goal of this placement is to pull the foot upward into dorsiflexion to retrain the muscle. There might be some inversion or eversion of the ankle (pulling inward or outward) depending on where your electrodes are placed, so adjust the placements if you are not getting a good dorsiflexion contraction.

THE HIP/PELVIS—GLUTEUS MEDIUS

Channels: 1

Method: EMS

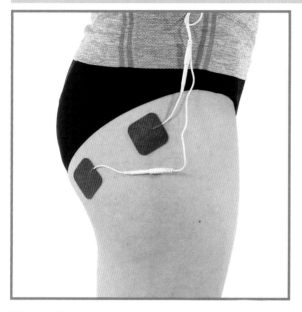

Place the electrodes along the gluteus medius muscle. This muscle helps abduct and medially rotate the hip. It's very important in keeping your hip stable when you are on one leg while walking and running. It also helps support the pelvis when walking or running.

The goal of this placement is to contract the gluteus medius to help retrain the muscle and stabilize the hip. You will feel it pulling your leg outward when it is contracting.

THE SHOULDER—DELTOID MUSCLES

Channels: 1

Method: EMS

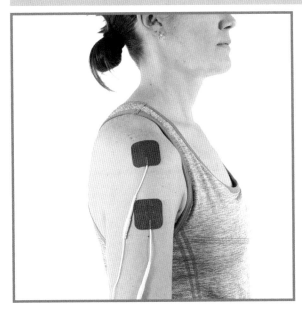

Place the electrodes along the middle deltoid muscle. Deltoid muscles consist of the anterior, middle, and posterior muscles. The middle deltoid muscles help you abduct or lift your arms out to the side. They also work with the rotator cuff muscles to help keep the shoulders stable.

The goal of this placement is to contract the middle deltoid muscle to help retrain the muscle and stabilize the shoulder. You will feel your arm pulling outward when it is contracting.

THE ELBOW/WRIST—WRIST EXTENSORS

Channels: 1

Method: EMS

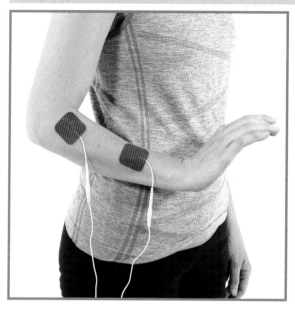

Place the electrodes along the wrist extensor muscles. These muscles help extend or lift up the wrist. They also help with wrist activities and attach at the lateral elbow. When it is irritated, it can cause tennis elbow.

The goal of this placement is to contract the wrist extensors to extend the wrist and help retrain the muscles at the elbow.

Chapter 8

Electrode Placements for Wireless Units

Unlike wired units that have two electrodes per channel, wireless units typically have one large electrode per channel. For a single-channel wireless TENS unit, place the electrode directly over, or just next to, the area of pain. For EMS, place it directly on the muscle you want to contract. For a two-channel TENS unit, place the two electrodes next to each other with the area of pain in the middle. For EMS, place the two electrodes along the muscle as you would with a wired unit.

Some wireless TENS units have two electrodes connected by a short wire for one channel. In this case, you would place the electrodes as you would for a wired unit, with the painful area in the middle of the two electrodes.

It is also possible to find a wireless TENS/EMS unit that uses two channels with four electrodes. In this case, the same rules for wired placements apply.

The placements for wireless electrodes on page 70 are all for TENS. You can use wireless for EMS, but make sure you are not crossing a joint or the spine (I do not recommend using EMS on your back or neck area for this reason). The rules for wired EMS units apply to the wireless units.

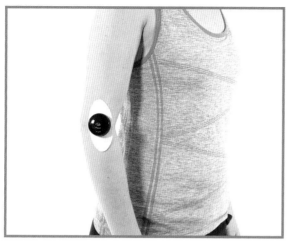

Elbow

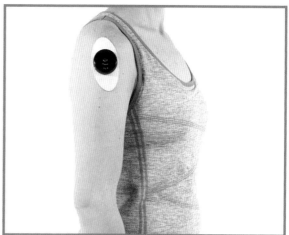

Shoulder

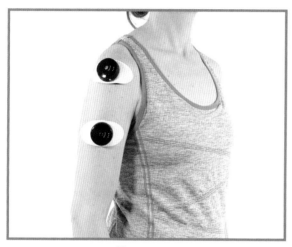

Upper arm

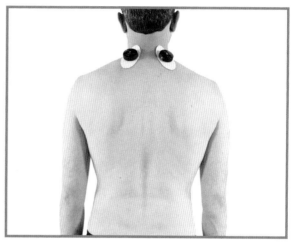

Neck

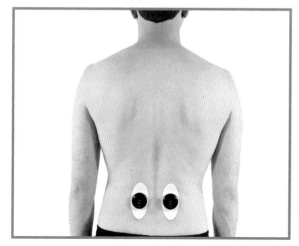

Lower back

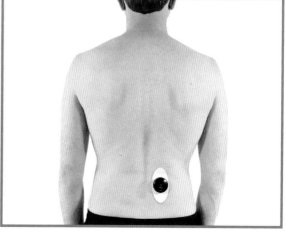

Lower back

Chapter 9

Stretches and Exercises with TENS and EMS

By now, I hope you know everything you ever wanted to know about TENS and EMS units. When used properly, they can be a great way to help relieve pain, improve circulation, and help the healing process. I want to take it one step further by showing you some very simple stretches and exercises you can do while you are using the TENS/EMS unit to help you get the best long-term pain relief. This will help improve your overall function and allow you to get back to doing the things you want to do.

Floor exercises can be performed on your bed or couch if you are unable to get on the floor. Also, the repetitions (reps) and sets (a group of repetitions) for each exercise or stretch are general starting points. How many you do depends on your particular injury (sprain, strain, tear, etc.) and how long you have had the injury (acute, subacute, chronic), so make sure to check with your doctor or physical therapist for the best number of reps (how many to do in one set), sets, and progression for your injury or ailment.

The placement of the electrodes for these exercises are general placements, but you can also use any of the placements shown in the previous chapters that work best for you. All of the placements below are for a TENS unit. Some of them can also be for EMS with placements shown in the previous chapters. I recommend using

EMS with isometric exercises so you are contracting the muscles but not moving the body part.

Quick note: with stretches and exercises, if you have time, working both sides is best. Often your good side is compensating for the painful side, and it will benefit from the treatment as well. This is especially important for the neck, back, and legs. When you do leg exercises while standing on the painful side, your muscles are getting a different workout (a closed-chain movement) than they get while you are standing on the good side and moving the painful side (an open-chain movement). So make sure you do both sides for the legs in particular. When working both sides, I like to alternate sides for each set. However, this is completely up to you, and if you want to do all the sets on one side and then switch, you can.

ISOMETRIC SIDE BEND

Reps: 5 | **Sets:** 2 | **Side:** Both | **Hold:** 3 to 5 seconds
Frequency: 2 to 3 times per day

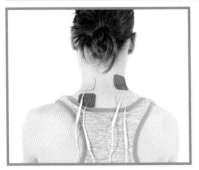 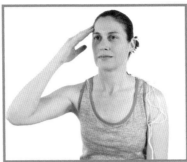 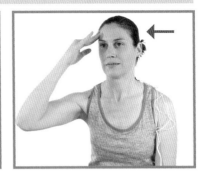

1. Place the electrodes in the way that works best for you. Start with your shoulders relaxed and your head in a neutral position. Place your hand on the side of your head you want to exercise to keep your head from actually moving.

2. Bend your head gently into your hand like you are trying to touch your ear to your shoulder.

ISOMETRIC ROTATION

Reps: 5 | **Sets:** 2 | **Side:** Both | **Hold:** 3 to 5 seconds
Frequency: 2 to 3 times per day

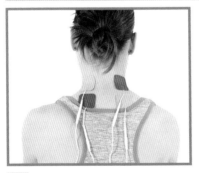 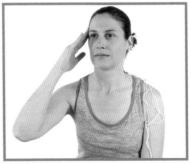 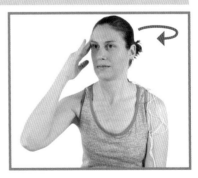

1. Place the electrodes in the way that works best for you. Start with your shoulders relaxed and your head in a neutral position. Place your hand on the side of your head you want to exercise to keep your head from actually moving.

2. Turn your head gently into your hand like you are trying to look behind you.

ISOMETRIC FLEXION

Reps: 5 | **Sets:** 2 | **Side:** Both | **Hold:** 3 to 5 seconds
Frequency: 2 to 3 times per day

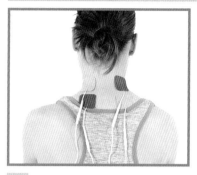 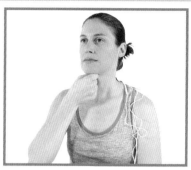 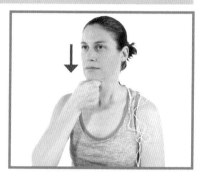

1. Place the electrodes in the way that works best for you. Start with your shoulders relaxed and your head in a neutral position. Place your hand in a fist under your chin to keep your head from actually moving.

2. Tilt your head gently down into your fist like you are trying to touch your chin to your chest.

ISOMETRIC EXTENSION

Reps: 5 | **Sets:** 2 | **Side:** Both | **Hold:** 3 to 5 seconds
Frequency: 2 to 3 times per day

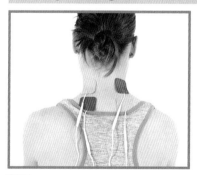 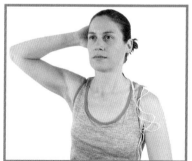 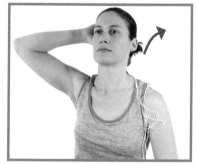

1. Place the electrodes in the way that works best for you. Start with your shoulders relaxed and your head in a neutral position. Place your hand on the back of your head to keep your head from actually moving.

2. Tilt your head gently into your hand like you are trying to look up toward the ceiling.

UPPER TRAPEZIUS STRETCH

Reps: 3 | **Sets:** 1 | **Side:** Both | **Hold:** 30 seconds
Frequency: 2 to 3 times per day

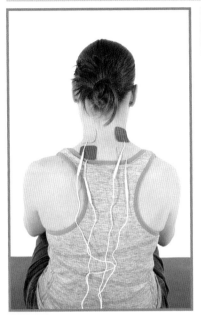 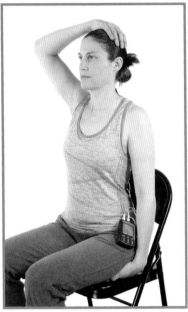 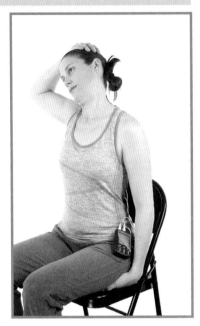

1. Place the electrodes in the way that works best for you. Sitting in a chair, place your hand on the side you want to stretch underneath your thigh so you are sitting on it. You can also place it behind your back. Place your other hand over your head on the side you want to stretch.

2. Gently pull toward the other side until you feel a stretch.

LEVATOR SCAPULAE STRETCH

Reps: 3 | **Sets:** 1 | **Side:** Both | **Hold:** 30 seconds
Frequency: 2 to 3 times per day

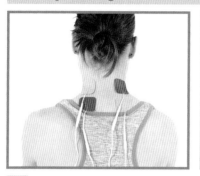 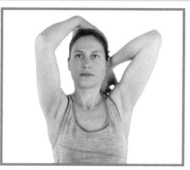 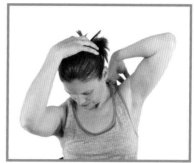

1. Place the electrodes in the way that works best for you. On the side you want to stretch, bring your arm up and place your hand on the back of your shoulder blade so your elbow is pointing upward toward the ceiling. Take your other hand over your head and place it on the back of your head.

2. Gently pull your head down at about a 45-degree angle, like you are pulling your nose toward your opposite knee until you feel a stretch.

ANTERIOR SCALENE STRETCH

Reps: 3 | **Sets:** 1 | **Side:** Both | **Hold:** 30 seconds
Frequency: 2 to 3 times per day

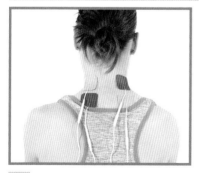 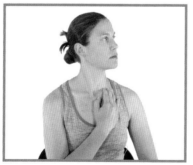 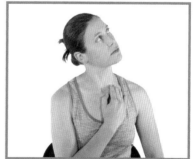

1. Place the electrodes in the way that works best for you. Place your opposite hand above the collarbone on the side you want to stretch and pull down gently. Turn your head toward the side you want to stretch.

2. While still pulling down, look up toward the ceiling.

PENDULUM CIRCLE

Reps: 10 | **Sets:** 2 to 3 | **Side:** Painful side

Frequency: 2 to 3 times per day

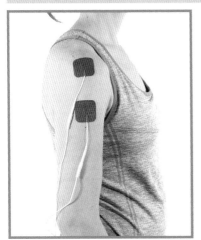 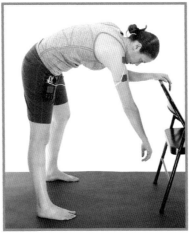 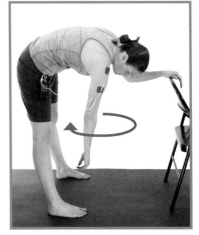

1. Place the electrodes in the way that works best for you. Use a sturdy chair or countertop to lean against. Hang your arm straight down toward the floor.

2. Move your body in a circle at your hips to make your arm move in a circular motion. Try not to actively move your arm.

TABLE SLIDES FLEXION

Reps: 10 | **Sets:** 2 to 3 | **Side:** Painful side | **Hold:** 1 to 2 seconds
Frequency: 2 to 3 times per day

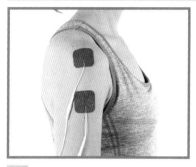 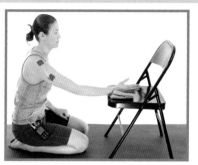 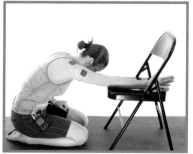

1. Place the electrodes in the way that works best for you. Sitting in front of a table or level surface, place your hand on the table with your thumb up. You can use a towel or blanket to help your hand slide.

2. Slide your arm forward as far as you comfortably can, and then slide back.

PULLEY

Reps: 10 | **Sets:** 2 to 3 | **Side:** Both | **Hold:** 1 to 2 seconds
Frequency: 2 to 3 times per day

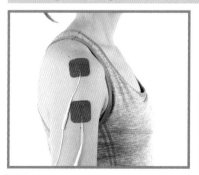 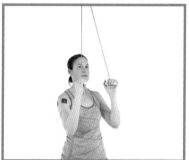 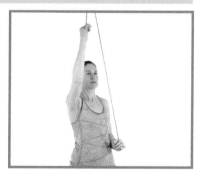

1. Place the electrodes in the way that works best for you. Hold onto the pulley system (or use a jump rope on a hook) with your thumbs pointing toward you, and try to relax the arm and shoulder of your painful side.

2. Gently pull down with the good side, bringing up the painful side without activating any muscles. Let gravity bring it back down, controlling it with the good side.

ISOMETRIC INTERNAL ROTATION

Reps: 5 | **Sets:** 2 | **Side:** Painful side | **Hold:** 3 to 5 seconds

Frequency: 2 to 3 times per day

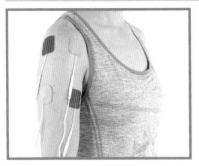 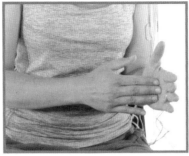 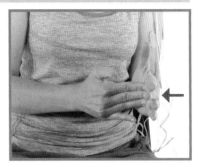

1. Place the electrodes in the way that works best for you. Sit or stand, then place your elbow by your side at about a 90-degree angle. Position your hand of the painful side with your thumb up and the other hand against the palm to prevent shoulder and arm movement.

2. Push your hand inward towards your body like you are going to place it on your stomach.

ISOMETRIC EXTERNAL ROTATION

Reps: 5 | **Sets:** 2 | **Side:** Painful side | **Hold:** 3 to 5 seconds

Frequency: 2 to 3 times per day

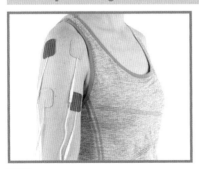 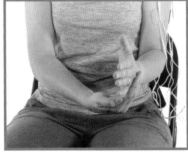 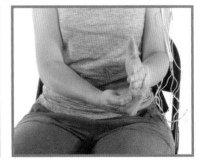

1. Place the electrodes in the way that works best for you. Sit or stand, then place your elbow by your side at about a 90-degree angle. Position your hand of the painful side with your thumb up and reach your other hand to the outside of the painful side to prevent shoulder and arm movement.

2. Push your hand away from your body, keeping your elbow by your side.

ISOMETRIC FLEXION

Reps: 5 | **Sets:** 2 | **Side:** Painful side | **Hold:** 3 to 5 seconds
Frequency: 2 to 3 times per day

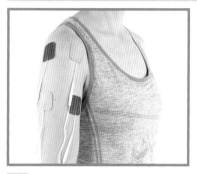 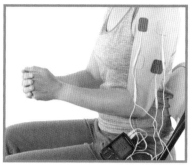 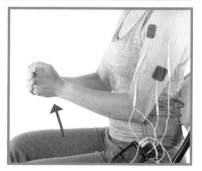

1. Place the electrodes in the way that works best for you. Sit or stand, then make a fist with your thumb facing upward on the painful side. Keep your elbow by your side at about a 90-degree angle. Place your other hand against the front of your fist to prevent shoulder movement.

2. Push forward and upward into your hand.

ISOMETRIC EXTENSION

Reps: 5 | **Sets:** 2 | **Side:** Painful side | **Hold:** 3 to 5 seconds
Frequency: 2 to 3 times per day

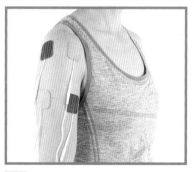 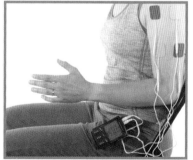 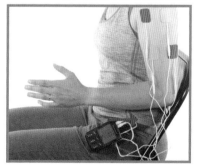

1. Place the electrodes in the way that works best for you. Sit in a chair, then place your elbow by your side at about a 90-degree angle. Position your hand on your painful side with your thumb facing upward.

2. Push your elbow backward into the chair and hold.

RESISTANCE BAND EXTERNAL ROTATION

Reps: 10 | **Sets:** 2 to 3 | **Hold:** 1 to 2 seconds
Frequency: 2 to 3 times per day

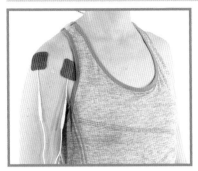 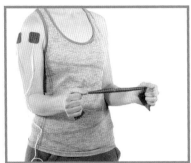 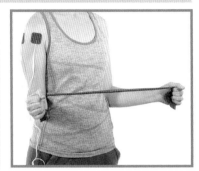

1. Place the electrodes in the way that works best for you. Hold a resistance band in front of you with your thumbs facing upward. Bend your elbows to about a 90-degree angle, and keep your elbows by your side.

2. Keeping your wrists in a neutral position, pull the band outward while keeping your elbows by your side. Slowly come back in.

RESISTANCE BAND SHOULDER FLEXION

Reps: 10 | **Sets:** 2 to 3 | **Side:** Painful side | **Hold:** 1 to 2 seconds
Frequency: 2 to 3 times per day

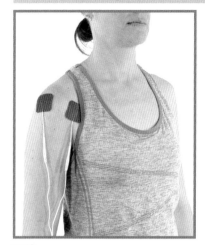 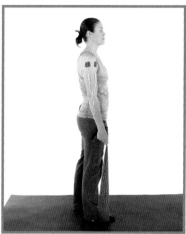 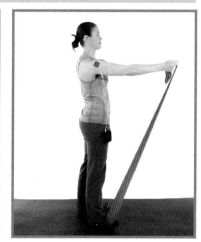

1. Place the electrodes in the way that works best for you. Anchor a resistance band underneath your foot on the side you are working. Turn your fist so your thumb is pointing forward.

2. Keeping your arm straight, raise your arm up to about 90 degrees, and slowly lower the band back down with a smooth movement.

RESISTANCE BAND SHOULDER EXTENSION

Reps: 10 | **Sets:** 2 to 3 | **Side:** Painful side | **Hold:** 1 to 2 seconds
Frequency: 2 to 3 times per day

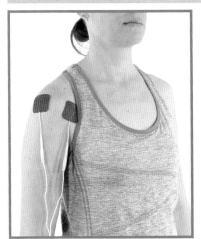 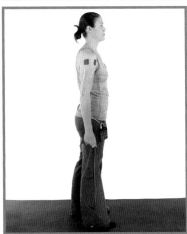 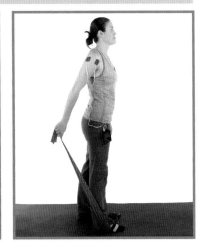

1. Place the electrodes in the way that works best for you. Anchor a resistance band underneath your foot on the side you are working. Turn your fist so your thumb is pointing forward.

2. Keeping your arm straight, pull your arm behind you to about 40 degrees, and slowly lower the band back down with a smooth movement.

ISOMETRIC ELBOW FLEXION (Biceps Curl)

Reps: 5 | **Sets:** 2 | **Side:** Painful side | **Hold:** 3 to 5 seconds
Frequency: 2 to 3 times per day

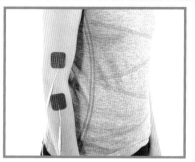 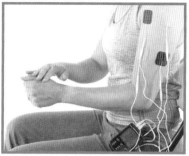 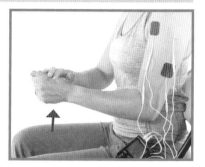

1. Place the electrodes in the way that works best for you. Sit or stand, then make a fist with your thumb facing upward on the hand with electrodes. Keep your elbow by your side at about a 90-degree angle. Place your other hand on top of that hand to prevent movement.

2. Push upward into your hand like you are doing a bicep curl.

ISOMETRIC ELBOW EXTENSION (Triceps Extension)

Reps: 5 | **Sets:** 2 | **Side:** Painful side | **Hold:** 3 to 5 seconds
Frequency: 2 to 3 times per day

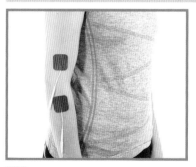 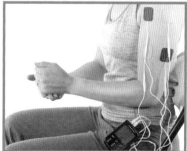 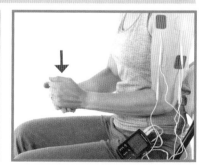

1. Place the electrodes in the way that works best for you. Sit or stand, then make a fist with your thumb facing upward on the hand with electrodes. Keep your elbow by your side at about a 90-degree angle. Place your other hand under that hand to prevent movement.

2. Push downward into your hand to activate the triceps muscles.

WRIST SUPINATION AND PRONATION

Reps: 10 | **Sets:** 2 to 3 | **Side:** Painful side | **Hold:** 1 to 2 seconds
Frequency: 2 to 3 times per day

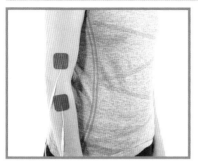 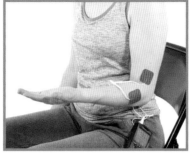 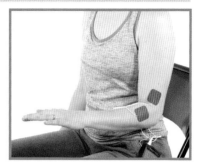

1. Place the electrodes in the way that works best for you. Keep the elbow on the painful side by your side, and bend it to about 90 degrees. Turn your wrist and forearm so your palm faces up (supination).

2. Keeping your elbow by your side, turn your palm to face down (pronation).

BICEPS STRETCH

Reps: 3 | **Sets:** 1 | **Side:** Painful side | **Hold:** 30 seconds
Frequency: 2 to 3 times per day

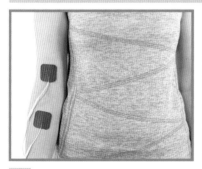 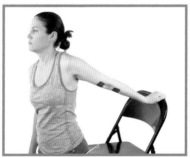 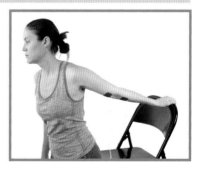

1. Place the electrodes in the way that works best for you. Keeping the arm and elbow as straight as possible on the painful side, grab onto something behind you like a table or chair.

2. Gently lean away from the table or chair until you feel a stretch.

RESISTANCE BAND BICEPS CURL

Reps: 10 | **Sets:** 2 to 3 | **Side:** Painful side | **Hold:** 1 to 2 seconds
Frequency: 2 to 3 times per day

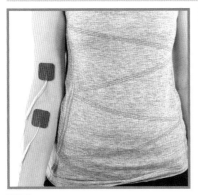 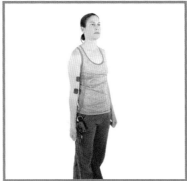 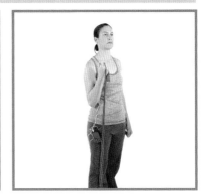

1. Place the electrodes in the way that works best for you. While standing, anchor down a resistance band with your foot. Hold the band in your hand of the painful side with your palm facing up and your elbow straight by your side.

2. Pull upward, bending at your elbow and keeping it by your side. Then slowly lower the band back down with a smooth movement.

TRICEPS STRETCH

Reps: 3 | **Sets:** 1 | **Side:** Painful side | **Hold:** 30 seconds
Frequency: 2 to 3 times per day

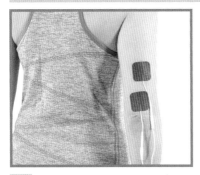 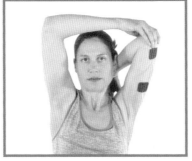 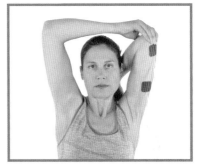

1. Place the electrodes in the way that works best for you. Bring the arm of your painful side up by your head, pointing your elbow up toward the ceiling.

2. Use your other hand to push or pull back behind you gently until you feel a stretch.

RESISTANCE BAND TRICEPS CURL

Reps: 10 | **Sets:** 2 to 3 | **Side:** Painful side | **Hold:** 1 to 2 seconds
Frequency: 2 to 3 times per day

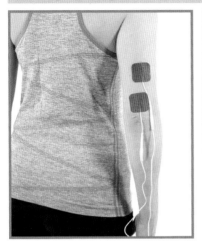 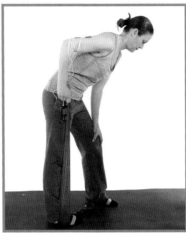 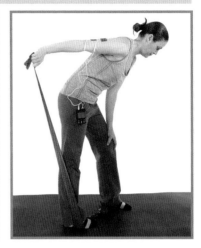

1. Place the electrodes in the way that works best for you. Stand up and bend slightly forward. Anchor a resistance band down with your foot. Hold the band in the hand of the painful side and put your elbow out behind you in a bent position.

2. Push the band behind you to straighten your elbow, and slowly lower the band back down with a smooth movement, bending your elbow again.

THORACIC SIDE BEND STRETCH

Reps: 3 | **Sets:** 1 | **Side:** Both | **Hold:** 10 to 15 seconds

Frequency: 2 to 3 times per day

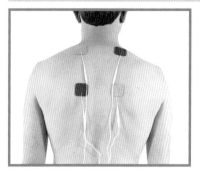 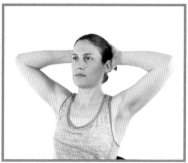 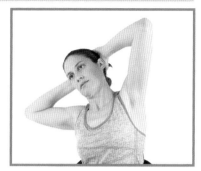

1. Place the electrodes in the way that works best for you. Place your hands on the back of your head with your elbows out.

2. Bend your upper body to the side, trying not to twist your body. Hold the stretch, and then repeat on the other side.

THORACIC ROTATION STRETCH

Reps: 5 | **Sets:** 2 | **Side:** Both | **Hold:** 10 to 15 seconds

Frequency: 2 to 3 times per day

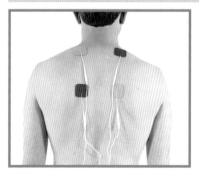 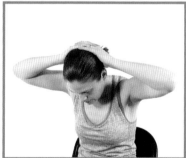 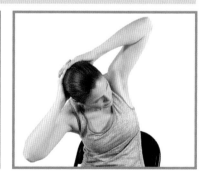

1. Place the electrodes in the way that works best for you. Place your hands behind your head with your elbows out. Bend your upper body slightly forward.

2. Rotate your upper body, bringing one elbow down toward your leg. Hold the stretch, and then repeat on the other side.

RHOMBOID STRETCH

Reps: 3 | **Sets:** 1 | **Hold:** 30 seconds

Frequency: 2 to 3 times per day

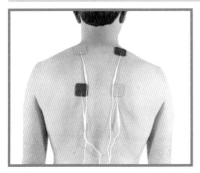 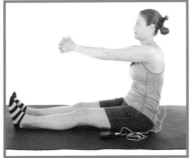 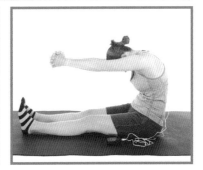

1. Place the electrodes in the way that works best for you. Sit on the floor with your legs straight out in front of you. Clasp your hands together in front of you with your elbows straight. (If you can't get in this position, you can also do it sitting in a chair, but you will not get as much of a stretch.)

2. Tuck your chin in toward your chest and push your clasped hands forward so you get an arch in your upper back.

THORACIC PRONE Y

Reps: 10 | **Sets:** 2 to 3 | **Side:** Both | **Hold:** 1 to 2 seconds

Frequency: 2 to 3 times per day

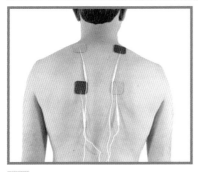 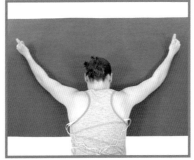 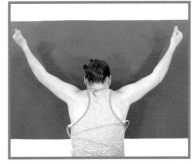

1. Place the electrodes in the way that works best for you. Lie on your stomach and put your arms out in front of you at an angle (like a Y) with your thumbs up.

2. Keeping them as straight as possible, raise your arms up off the floor (or bed) while squeezing your shoulder blades together.

THORACIC PRONE T

Reps: 10 | **Sets:** 2 to 3 | **Side:** Both | **Hold:** 1 to 2 seconds
Frequency: 2 to 3 times per day

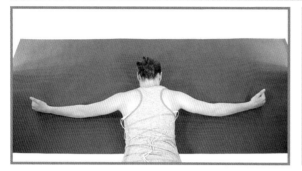 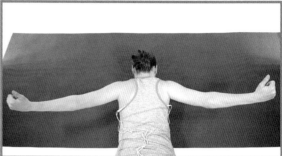

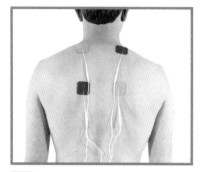

1. Place the electrodes in the way that works best for you. Lie on your stomach and put your arms straight out to the side (like a T) with your thumbs up.

2. Keeping them as straight as possible, raise your arms up off the floor (or bed) while squeezing your shoulder blades together.

THORACIC PRONE W

Reps: 10 | **Sets:** 2 to 3 | **Side:** Both | **Hold:** 1 to 2 seconds
Frequency: 2 to 3 times per day

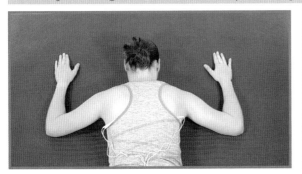 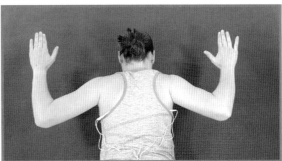

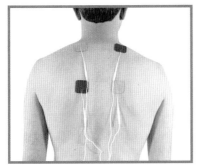

1. Place the electrodes in the way that works best for you. Lie on your stomach and put your arms out to the side with your elbows bent (like a W) and your palms down.

2. Raise your arms up off the floor (or bed) while squeezing your shoulder blades together.

PRAYER STRETCH/CHILD'S POSE STRETCH

Reps: 3 | **Sets:** 1 | **Hold:** 30 seconds

Frequency: 2 to 3 times per day

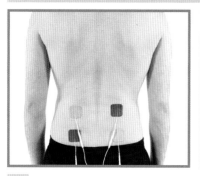
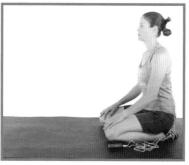
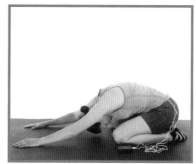

1. Place the electrodes in the way that works best for you. Sit back on your feet (or as far as you can comfortably go) with the top of your feet on the floor (or bed).

2. With you head down, stretch your arms out in front of you, sliding them on the floor (or bed) as far as you can.

CAT/DOG (Cat/Cow) STRETCH

Reps: 5 | **Sets:** 2 | **Hold:** 3 to 5 seconds

Frequency: 2 to 3 times per day

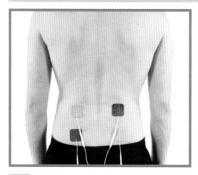
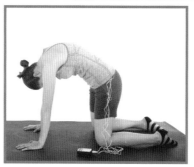
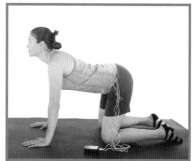

1. Place the electrodes in the way that works best for you. Get on all fours in the quadruped position. Arch your back like a cat and tuck your chin in to your chest at the same time.

2. Drop your back down into a sagging (or saddle) position and pick your head up, looking straight ahead.

SUPINE TRUNK ROTATION STRETCH

Reps: 3 | **Sets:** 1 | **Side:** Both | **Hold:** 30 seconds

Frequency: 2 to 3 times per day

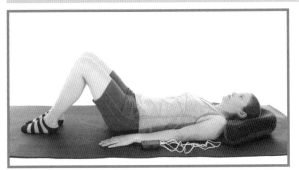 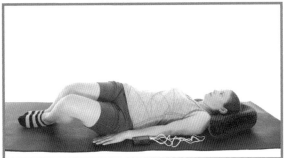

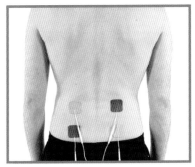

1. Place the electrodes in the way that works best for you. Lie on the floor (or bed) with your knees bent and your feet close together.

2. Keeping your upper back on the floor, rotate your knees to one side as far as you comfortably can.

PELVIC TILT

Reps: 10 | **Sets:** 2 to 3 | **Hold:** 3 to 5 seconds

Frequency: 2 to 3 times per day

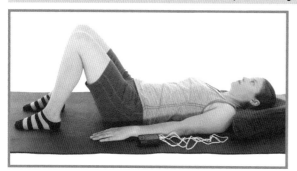 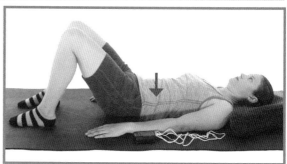

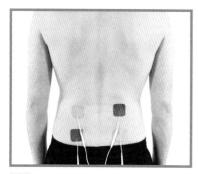

1. Place the electrodes in the way that works best for you. Lie down on your back with your knees bent.

2. Flatten your back by rotating your pelvis backward. Imagine someone has their hand under the curve of your back, and you are trying to push down on it with your back, not with your legs or by lifting your buttocks.

BRIDGE

Reps: 10 | **Sets:** 2 to 3 | **Hold:** 1 to 2 seconds

Frequency: 2 to 3 times per day

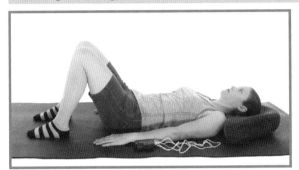
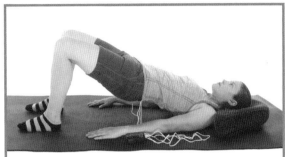

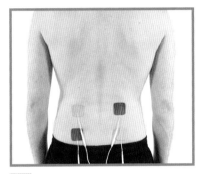

1. Place the electrodes in the way that works best for you. Lie on your back with your knees bent and your feet flat on the floor (or bed).

2. With your arms by your side, push your hips up off the floor until you make a straight line with your body, and then slowly come back down.

Try to roll your back when coming up and down, like you are moving one segment of your back at a time in a smooth motion.

HIP FLEXOR STRETCH

Reps: 3 | **Sets:** 1 | **Side:** Both | **Hold:** 30 seconds
Frequency: 2 to 3 times per day

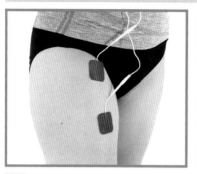 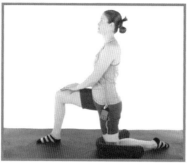 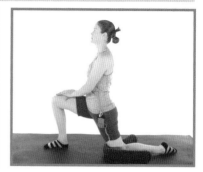

1. Place the electrodes in the way that works best for you. Start off in a lunge position with your knee on the side you want to stretch on the floor. Use a pillow under your knee if you would like.

2. Keeping your back straight and upright, lean forward until you feel a stretch.

SEATED HIP FLEXION

Reps: 10 | **Sets:** 2 to 3 | **Side:** Both | **Hold:** 1 to 2 seconds
Frequency: 2 to 3 times per day

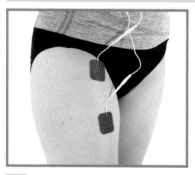 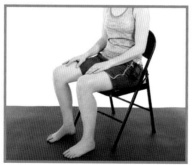 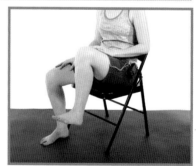

1. Place the electrodes in the way that works best for you. Sit in a chair with your back straight and your feet flat on the floor.

2. Lift your knee up toward the ceiling without leaning back. Then, slowly bring it back down.

HAMSTRING STRETCH

Reps: 3 | **Sets:** 1 | **Side:** Both | **Hold:** 30 seconds
Frequency: 2 to 3 times per day

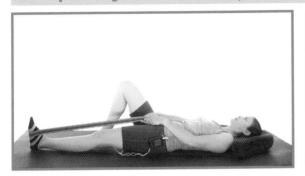 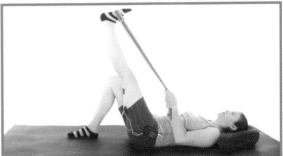

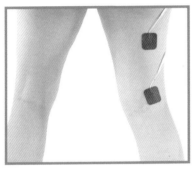

1. Place the electrodes in the way that works best for you. Lie on your back and place a strap, belt, or dog leash around the ball of your foot. You can bend the knee of the leg you are not stretching to help relax your back.

2. Keeping your knee straight, pull your leg up with the strap until you feel a stretch behind your knee/leg.

If your knee bends when you are bringing it up, come back down enough to be able to keep the knee straight. Keeping the knee/leg straight through the whole movement will give you the best stretch.

ILIOTIBIAL (IT) BAND STRETCH

Reps: 3 | **Sets:** 1 | **Side:** Both | **Hold:** 30 seconds
Frequency: 2 to 3 times per day

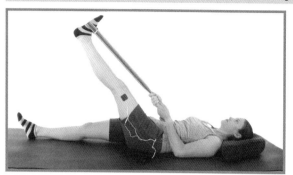 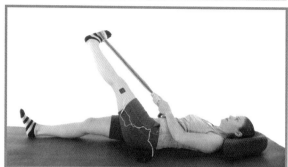

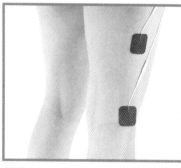

1. Place the electrodes in the way that works best for you. Lie on your back and place a strap, belt, or dog leash around the ball of your foot. Pull your leg up, keeping your knee straight.

2. When you start to feel a slight stretch, pull your leg across your body until you feel a stretch on the outside of your leg.

CALF STRETCH (Runner's Stretch)

Reps: 3 | **Sets:** 1 | **Side:** Both | **Hold:** 30 seconds
Frequency: 2 to 3 times per day

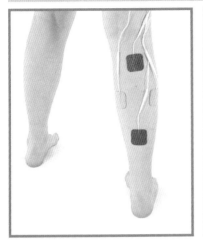 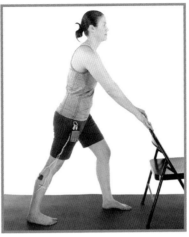 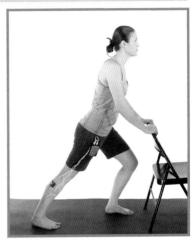

1. Place the electrodes in the way that works best for you. Using a chair, wall, or something sturdy for balance, stand with one foot (the side you want to stretch) directly behind you and the other in front in a lunge position. Keep your back heel down and your feet facing forward.

2. With your back leg straight, bend your front knee forward until you feel a stretch in your back leg/calf area (the back heel should stay down the whole time).

HEEL RAISE

Reps: 10 | **Sets:** 2 to 3 | **Hold:** 1 to 2 seconds
Frequency: 2 to 3 times per day

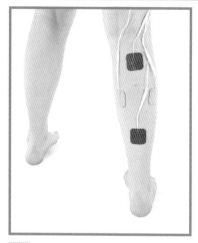 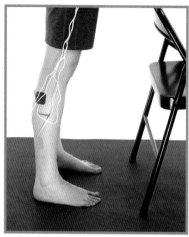 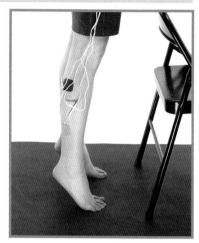

1. Place the electrodes in the way that works best for you. With your feet about shoulder-width apart, stand behind a sturdy chair or countertop and hold on for balance.

2. Lift your heels off the floor as high as you can, and slowly come back down.

STRAIGHT LEG RAISE (SLR)

Reps: 10 | **Sets:** 2 to 3 | **Side:** Both | **Hold:** 1 to 2 seconds
Frequency: 2 to 3 times per day

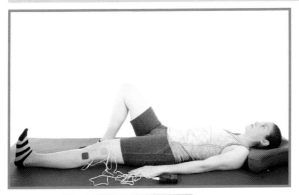
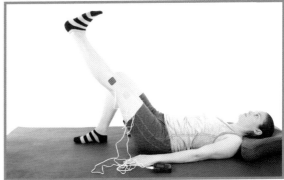
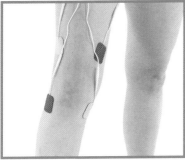

1. Place the electrodes in the way that works best for you. Lie down on your back with your good knee bent upward. Straighten out the leg with electrodes. Pull your toes toward you to lock your knee.

2. Keeping your knee straight, lift the leg to the height of the other, and slowly come back down.

QUAD SET

Reps: 10 | **Sets:** 2 | **Side:** Painful Side | **Hold:** 3 to 5 seconds
Frequency: 2 to 3 times per day

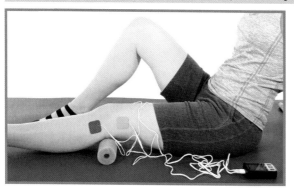 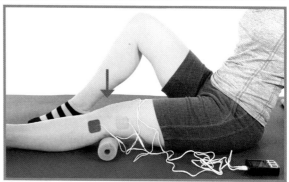

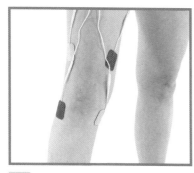

1. Place the electrodes in the way that works best for you. Sit on the floor (or bed) with the leg on your painful side straight out in front of you. Place a rolled-up towel or foam roller under your knee.

2. Push your knee down into the towel or foam roller, and try to keep your heel on the floor.

SEATED KNEE EXTENSION/LONG ARC QUAD (LAQ)

Reps: 10 | **Sets:** 2 to 3 | **Side:** Both | **Hold:** 1 to 2 seconds
Frequency: 2 to 3 times per day

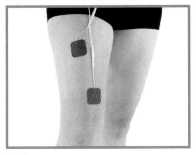 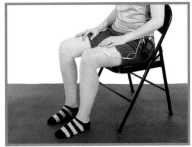 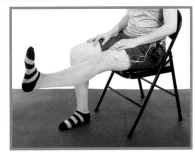

1. Place the electrodes in the way that works best for you. Sit in a chair, keeping your back straight.

2. Extend your leg straight out while pulling your toes toward you at the end of the movement. Slowly come back down.

CLAMSHELL

Reps: 10 | **Sets:** 2 to 3 | **Side:** Painful side | **Hold:** 1 to 2 seconds
Frequency: 2 to 3 times per day

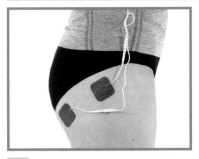 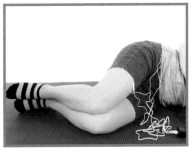 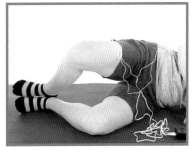

1. Place the electrodes in the way that works best for you. Lie on your side with your painful side up and your knees bent forward so your heels are aligned with your body.

2. Keeping your body/hips perpendicular to the floor (or bed) and without rotating your hips back, lift the top knee toward the ceiling while keeping your feet together. Slowly come back down.

ANKLE PUMP

Reps: 10 | **Sets:** 2 to 3 | **Side:** Both | **Hold:** 1 to 2 seconds
Frequency: 2 to 3 times per day

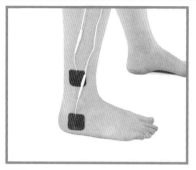 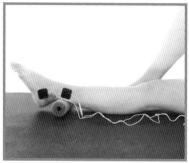 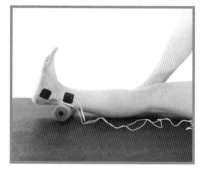

1. Place the electrodes in the way that works best for you. Extend the leg of the side with electrodes straight out in front of you. Place a roll or towel just under your ankle so your heel can move freely. Push your foot down like you are pushing on a pedal (plantar flexion).

2. Pull your foot up toward you (dorsiflexion).

PLANTAR FLEXION WITH RESISTANCE BAND

Reps: 10 | **Sets:** 2 to 3 | **Side:** Both | **Hold:** 1 to 2 seconds
Frequency: 2 to 3 times per day

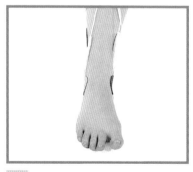 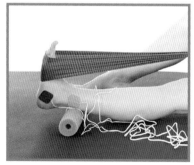 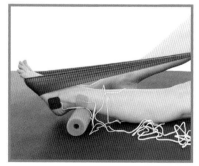

1. Place the electrodes in the way that works best for you. Extend the leg of the side with electrodes out in front of you, placing a roll just under your ankle so your heel can move freely. Place a resistance band around the ball of your foot.

2. Push your foot down like you are pushing on a pedal.

DORSIFLEXION WITH RESISTANCE BAND

Reps: 10 | **Sets:** 2 to 3 | **Side:** Both | **Hold:** 1 to 2 seconds

Frequency: 2 to 3 times per day

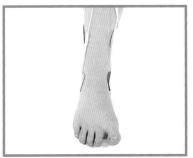 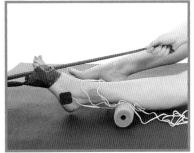 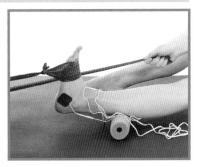

1. Place the electrodes in the way that works best for you. Extend the leg of the side with electrodes out in front of you, placing a roll just under your ankle so your heel can move freely. Place a resistance band around the top of your foot, and wrap the band around something in front of you or have someone hold the band in front of you.

2. Pull your toes up toward you.

EVERSION WITH RESISTANCE BAND

Reps: 10 | **Sets:** 2 to 3 | **Side:** Both | **Hold:** 1 to 2 seconds

Frequency: 2 to 3 times per day

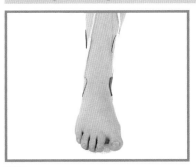 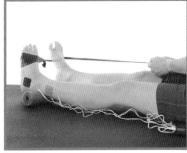 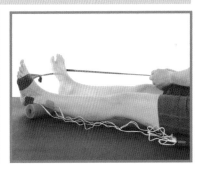

1. Place the electrodes in the way that works best for you. Extend your legs out in front of you, placing a roll just under the ankle with electrodes so your heel can move freely. Place a resistance band around the ball of your foot with electrodes, and wrap the band around your other foot for an anchor.

2. Just at your ankle, pull outward, away from the other foot.

INVERSION WITH RESISTANCE BAND

Reps: 10 | **Sets:** 2 to 3 | **Side:** Both | **Hold:** 1 to 2 seconds

Frequency: 2 to 3 times per day

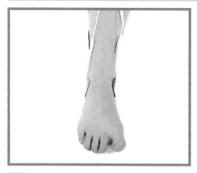 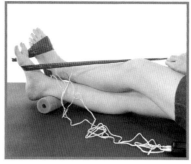 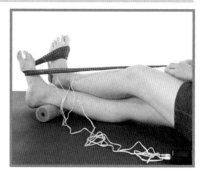

1. Place the electrodes in the way that works best for you. Extend your legs out in front of you, crossing the leg of the side with electrodes over the other leg. Place a resistance band around the ball of your foot on the painful side, and wrap the band around the other foot for an anchor.

2. Just at your ankle, pull the side you are exercising away from the other foot.

BALL/FOAM ROLL/FROZEN BOTTLE ROLL

Reps: 10 | **Sets:** 2 to 3 | **Side:** Painful side | **Hold:** 1 to 2 seconds

Frequency: 2 to 3 times per day

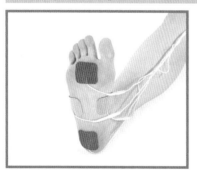 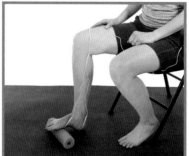 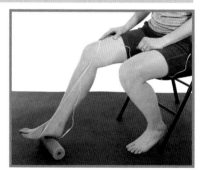

1. Place the electrodes in the way that works best for you. Sit in a chair, and place a foam roll or frozen water bottle under your painful foot. You can also use a tennis, massage, or lacrosse ball.

2. Start with the roll (or ball) at the ball of your foot. Roll it down to your heel, and then back to the ball of your foot.

Conclusion

You should now have a good idea of how to use a TENS/EMS unit, what kind of unit will work best for you, and some stretches and exercises to use in conjunction with the unit to get the best possible results.

Remember, there is a learning curve to using the units, and placements are not always exact. You will benefit from placements depending on your body type, size, and reaction to the treatment. Try not to get frustrated if you don't get it exactly right the first few times you try it.

If you are interested in seeing videos of more stretches and exercises for injuries and ailments of all kinds—or if you just want to say hi to the pups and me—make sure to stop by my website (AskDoctorJo.com) and my YouTube channel (youtube.com/AskDoctorJo). You can also find me on social media under the handle AskDoctorJo on Facebook, Pinterest, Twitter, and Instagram.

And remember, be safe, have fun, and I hope you feel better soon!

References

Balagué, F., A. F. Mannion, F. Pellisé, et al. "Non-specific Low Back Pain." *Lancet* 379, no. 9814 (February 4, 2012):482–491. https://doi.org/10.1016/S0140-6736(11)60610-7.

Franco, O.S., F. S. Paulitsch, A. P. Pereira AP, et al. "Effects of Different Frequencies of Transcutaneous Electrical Nerve Stimulation on Venous Vascular Reactivity." *Brazilian Journal of Medical and Biological Research* 47, no. 5 (2014):411–8.

Electrotherapy. "Transcutaneous Electrical Nerve Stimulation (TENS)." Accessed April 26, 2019. http://www.electrotherapy.org/modality/transcutaneous-electrical-nerve-stimulation-tens.

ExcelHealth, Inc. "The History of Electrotherapy." Accessed March 16, 2019. https://www.ireliev.com/wp-content/uploads/2017/01/The-History-of-Electrotherapy-1.pdf.

Johnson, M. "Transcutaneous Electrical Nerve Stimulation: Mechanisms, Clinical Application and Evidence." *Reviews in Pain* 1, no. 1 (2007):7–11.

Karasuno, H., H. Ogihara, K. Morishita, et al. "The Combined Effects of Transcutaneous Electrical Nerve Stimulation (TENS) and Stretching on Muscle Hardness and Pressure Pain Threshold." *Journal of Physical Therapy Science* 28, no. 4 (2016): 1124–30.

Katz, J. and B. N. Rosenbloom. "The Golden Anniversary of Melzack and Wall's Gate Control Theory of Pain: Celebrating 50 Years of Pain Research and Management." *Pain Research and Management* 20, no. 6 (2015):285–6.

LeFort, S., L. Webster, K. Lorig, et al. *Living a Healthy Life with Chronic Pain*. Boulder, CO: Bull Publishing Company, 2015.

Mendell, L. M. "Constructing and Deconstructing the Gate Theory of Pain." *Pain* 155, no. 2 (2013):210–6.

Nnoaham, K. E. and J. Kumbang. "Transcutaneous Electrical Nerve Stimulation (TENS) for Chronic Pain." *Cochrane Database of Systematic Reviews* 3, no. CD003222 (2008). https://doi.org10.1002/14651858.CD003222.pub2.

Rennie, S. "Electrophysical Agents—Contraindications and Precautions: An Evidence-Based Approach to Clinical Decision Making in Physical Therapy." *Physiotherapy Canada* 62, no. 5 (2011):1–80.

Vance C. G., D. L. Dailey, B. A. Rakel BA, et al. "Using TENS for Pain Control: The State of the Evidence." *Pain Management* 4, no. 3 (2014):197–209.

Wall, P. D. and W. H. Sweet. "Temporary Abolition of Pain in Man." *Science* 155 (January 6, 1967):108–109.

Zhang, J. M. and J. An. "Cytokines, Inflammation, and Pain." *International Anesthesiology Clinics* 45, no. 2 (2007):27–37.